Rapid Cardiac Care

Rapid Cardiac Care

Emma Menzies-Gow
Senior Lecturer – Cardiac Care
Kingston University and St George's, University of London, UK

Christine Spiers
Principal Lecturer – Cardiac Care
School of Health Sciences, University of Brighton, UK

WILEY Blackwell

Registered Office(s)
John Wiley & Sons, Inc., 111 River Street, Hoboken, NJ 07030, USA
John Wiley & Sons Ltd, The Atrium, Southern Gate, Chichester, West Sussex, PO19 8SQ, UK

Editorial Office
9600 Garsington Road, Oxford, OX4 2DQ, UK

For details of our global editorial offices, customer services, and more information about Wiley products visit us at www.wiley.com.

Wiley also publishes its books in a variety of electronic formats and by print-on-demand. Some content that appears in standard print versions of this book may not be available in other formats.

Library of Congress Cataloging-in-Publication Data

Names: Menzies-Gow, Emma, author. | Spiers, Christine, author.
Title: Rapid cardiac care / by Emma Menzies-Gow, Christine Spiers.
Description: Hoboken, NJ : Wiley, 2017. | Includes index. |
Identifiers: LCCN 2017030441 (print) | LCCN 2017030987 (ebook) | ISBN 9781119220282 (pdf) |
   ISBN 9781119220343 (epub) | ISBN 9781119220275 (paper)
Subjects: | MESH: Cardiovascular Diseases–therapy | Acute Disease–therapy | Cardiovascular
   Diseases–diagnosis | Diagnostic Techniques, Cardiovascular
Classification: LCC RC667 (ebook) | LCC RC667 (print) | NLM WG 166 | DDC 616.1–dc23
LC record available at https://lccn.loc.gov/2017030441

Cover Design: Wiley
Cover Image: © Caiaimage/Sam Edwards/Gettyimages

Set in 9.5/11.5pt Frutiger Light by SPi Global, Pondicherry, India
Printed and bound in Malaysia by Vivar Printing Sdn Bhd

10 9 8 7 6 5 4 3 2 1

Dedication

Heidi Simpson (née Clinton)

This book is dedicated to our much loved friend Heidi, an outstanding nurse whose contribution to healthcare education has influenced the clinical practice of many nurses and practitioners working in acute and intensive care

Contents

List of Abbreviations

ABGs   Arterial blood gases
ACE-I   Angiotensin-converting-enzyme inhibitors
ACLS   Advanced Cardiac Life Support
ACS   Acute coronary syndromes
AED   Automated external defibrillator
AF   Atrial fibrillation
ALP   Alkaline phosphatase
ALT   Alanine transaminase
APTT   Activated partial thromboplastin time
ARB   Angiotensin receptor blocker
ARVC   Arrhythmogenic right ventricular cardiomyopathy
AS   Aortic stenosis
AST   Aspartate transaminase
AV   Atrio-ventricular
AVNRT   A-V nodal re-entry tachycardia
AVRT   A-V re-entry tachycardia
BBB   Bundle branch block
BNP   B-type natriuretic peptides
BP   Blood pressure
bpm   beats per minute
CCBs   Calcium channel blockers
CK-MB   Creatinine kinase myocardial isoenzyme
CMR   Cardiac magnetic resonance
COPD   Chronic obstructive pulmonary disease
CPAP   Continuous positive airway pressure
CPR   Cardiopulmonary resuscitation
CRP   C-reactive protein
CRT   Cardiac resynchronisation therapy
CRT-D   Cardiac resynchronisation therapy – defibrillator
CRT-P   Cardiac resynchronisation therapy – pacemaker
CT   Computed tomography
CXR   Chest X-ray
DCCV   Direct current cardioversion
DCM   Dilated cardiomyopathy
ECG   Electrocardiogram
EDV   end diastolic volume
eGFR   Estimated glomerular filtration rate
ESR   Erythrocyte sedimentation rate
FBC   Full blood count
GTN   Glyceryl trinitrate
HbA1c   Glycated haemoglobin
HCM   Hypertrophic cardiomyopathy

HF	Heart failure
HF-PEF	Heart failure with Preserved Ejection Fraction
HF-REF	Heart failure with Reduced Ejection Fraction
ICD	Implantable cardioverter defibrillator
IE	Infective endocarditis
JVD	Jugular venous distension
LAD	Left anterior descending coronary artery
LAFB	Left anterior fascicular block
LBB	Left bundle branch
LBBB	Left bundle branch block
LCx	Left circumflex
LDL	Low-density lipoproteins
LMWH	Low molecular weight heparin
LPFB	Left posterior fascicular block
LQTS	Long QT syndrome
LV	Left ventricle
LVEDP	Left ventricular end diastolic pressure
LVEDV	Left ventricular end diastolic volume
LVF	Left ventricular failure
LVH	Left ventricular hypertrophy
LVOT	Left ventricular outflow tract
mV	millivolts
MR	Mitral regurgitation
NOAC	Non-vitamin K oral anti-coagulant
NSAIDs	Non-steroidal anti-inflammatory drugs
NSTEMI	Non ST-segment elevation myocardial infarction
NT-proBNP	N-terminal prohormone of brain natriuretic peptide
NYHA	New York Heart Association
PA	Posterior-anterior
P-PCI	Primary percutaneous coronary intervention
PCI	Percutaneous coronary intervention
PDA	Posterior descending artery
PEA	Pulseless electrical activity
PMH	Past medical history
PVCs	Premature ventricular contractions
QTc	Corrected QT
RAAS	Renin-angiotensin-aldosterone system
RBB	Right bundle branch
RBBB	Right bundle branch block
RCA	Right coronary artery
RV	Right ventricle
RVH	Right ventricular hypertrophy
RVOT	Right ventricular outflow tract
SA	Sino-atrial (node)
SCN5A	Sodium channel gene 5A

STEMI	ST-segment elevation myocardial infarction
SVT	Supraventricular tachycardia
TAVI	Transcutaneous aortic valve implantation
TEVAR	Thoracic endovascular aortic repair
TOE	Trans-oesophageal echocardiogram
TC	Takotsubo cardiomyopathy
TOE	Transoesophageal echocardiogram
TTE	Trans-thoracic echocardiogram
UA	Unstable angina
U&E	Urea and electrolytes
UFH	Unfractionated heparin
VF	Ventricular fibrillation
VT	Ventricular tachycardia
WPW	Wolff-Parkinson-White

Preface

Many cardiac conditions present suddenly, requiring a rapid response from healthcare practitioners. 'Rapid Cardiac Care' provides a concise text to guide the assessment and management of patients experiencing a variety of cardiac conditions. A systematic approach has been used to structure your assessment of the patient data and to prioritise management interventions. An overview of cardiac anatomy and physiology precedes sections on cardiac assessment, investigations, history taking, physical examination, symptom review and cardiac rhythm evaluation. The 12-lead ECG is a pivotal investigation in the evaluation of many cardiac conditions and therefore a tool to guide rapid interpretation is also provided. The care of patients with a range of cardiac conditions is presented in an A–Z format, which will direct the reader straight to the relevant sections.

Acknowledgements

We would like to thank the team at Wiley for their assistance throughout the production of this book.

Sincere thanks are extended to our families, for their constant support, patience and encouragement. We would especially like to acknowledge our fathers who influenced our lives immensely.

Part 1 Cardiac Anatomy and Physiology

Anatomy

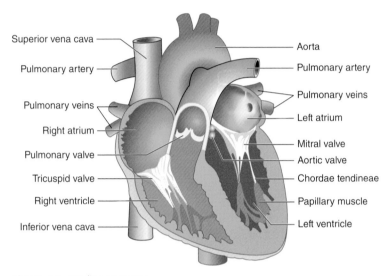

Superior vena cava

Pulmonary artery

Pulmonary veins

Right atrium

Pulmonary valve

Tricuspid valve

Right ventricle

Inferior vena cava

Aorta

Pulmonary artery

Pulmonary veins

Left atrium

Mitral valve

Aortic valve

Chordae tendineae

Papillary muscle

Left ventricle

Figure 1.1 Cardiac anatomy.

The heart is a cone-shaped, muscular organ with four chambers that propel blood through the circulatory system (Figure 1.1). The two upper chambers, the atria, and the ventricles below are separated by the annulus fibrosus (AV ring), a layer of connective tissue that forms the cardiac skeleton, seen on the external surface of the heart as the atrio-ventricular (AV) groove. The mitral and tricuspid (AV) valves and aortic and pulmonary (semilunar) valves form part of the AV ring. Each valve consists of two or three cusps arising from an annulus. Healthy valves maintain forward blood flow through the heart, opening and closing in response to changes in pressure between the chambers. The interatrial septum separates the two atria; the ventricles are separated by the interventricular septum, which is visible on the outside of the heart as anterior-posterior interventricular groove.

The heart wall is formed from three layers of tissue that provide different functions. The external layer is the pericardium, which surrounds the heart and the roots of the aorta and pulmonary arterial trunk. It consists of two distinct layers: the outermost fibrous layer and serous layer beneath. The serous pericardium has a visceral layer, known as the epicardium, which surrounds the myocardium and doubles back on itself to form the parietal pericardium, which lines the tough, outer fibrous layer. The space between the two layers contains a small volume of fluid to reduce friction during myocardial contraction. The central, thickest layer of the heart wall is the myocardium. It contains clusters of cardiac muscle cells known as myocytes, each surrounded by connective tissue and a network of capillaries. The internal surface of the heart is lined with a single, continuous layer of endothelial cells known as the endocardium. This facilitates smooth blood flow through the chambers and across the valves and provides some protection from the formation of thrombi.

Cardiac cycle

Cardiac output is the volume of blood ejected from the left ventricle (LV) in one minute, i.e. heart rate × stroke volume. It is approximately 4–7 L/min. The cardiac conduction system controls heart rate variability and co-ordinated systolic (contraction) and diastolic (relaxation and filling) activity of the cardiac chambers to maximise cardiac output.

The superior and inferior vena cava empty into the right atrium, enabling the return of deoxygenated blood to the heart. The coronary sinus, a large cardiac vein, also drains deoxygenated blood from the myocardium into the right atrium. The tricuspid valve opens to permit blood to enter the right ventricle (RV); atrial contraction provides extra force to expel blood from the chamber, known as the 'atrial kick', to optimise the end diastolic volume (EDV) of the ventricles.

During systole, the three papillary muscles in the RV contract, tightening the chordae tendineae, attached to the cusps of the tricuspid valve to ensure the valve leaflets remain closed, preventing regurgitation of blood into the right atrium. Pressure within the RV will rise until it exceeds the pressure within the pulmonary circulation beyond, forcing the pulmonary valve to open and blood to flow into the pulmonary arterial trunk. During ventricular diastole, the pulmonary arteries will rapidly recoil to enable blood to fall back towards the RV, closing the pulmonary valve.

Having completed gaseous exchange within the alveoli and pulmonary capillaries, oxygenated blood returns to the left atrium via four pulmonary veins. The increase in pressure within the atrial chamber forces the mitral valve to open and ventricular filling to begin. During diastole, the ventricular myocytes will stretch to accommodate the volume of blood, which directly correlates with the force of contraction that occurs during systolic contraction (Frank Starling's Law). The two papillary muscles contract first, once systole begins, tightening the chordae tendineae attached to the two cusps of the mitral valve to prevent regurgitation. The LV and septum then contract to increase the pressure (preload) within the LV. Once the preload pressure exceeds the pressure in the aorta beyond the aortic valve (afterload), blood will leave the LV, referred to as the stroke volume, crossing the aortic valve into the aorta to supply the arterial circulation. The term 'ejection fraction' refers to the stroke volume as a percentage of the left ventricular EDV (LVEDV), usually approximately 60–70% at rest. As systole ends, diastole begins again and a small volume of blood in the aorta will return towards the LV, closing the aortic valve cusps and simultaneously perfusing the coronary arteries originating at the aortic root.

Cardiac conduction system

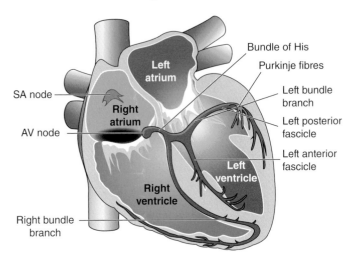

Figure 1.2 Cardiac conduction system.

The cardiac conduction system lies beneath the endocardium within the myocardium and consists of specialised myocytes responsible for generating and transmitting an impulse across the heart (Figure 1.2). The sino-atrial (SA) node, located on the posterior wall of the right atrium, is the primary pacemaker of the heart and therefore determines heart rate. It is capable of regular spontaneous depolarisation without external stimulus. However, the autonomic nervous system controls the SA nodal firing rate, permitting heart rate variability in response to fluctuating metabolic demand. Increased sympathetic activity will cause an increase in the SA nodal firing rate, for example during exercise. The heart rate is slowed via the vagus nerve, part of the parasympathetic nervous system.

Transition cells surrounding the SA node transfer the impulse across to the surrounding atrial myocytes, which in turn propagate the impulse to the remaining atrial cells, causing depolarisation and contraction. The annulus fibrosus, or AV ring, prevents direct transmission of the impulse to the ventricle. In response to atrial stimulation, the AV node transmits the impulse to the ventricular myocardium via the His-Purkinje system. After leaving the AV node, the impulse traverses the Bundle of His, which divides into two bundle branch systems. The right bundle branch is a thin, long strand, which runs down the right side of the interventricular septum and supplies conduction to the RV. The left bundle branch comprises shorter, thicker fibres, which divide into two branches called fascicles. The left anterior fascicle is the thinner of the two fascicles and supplies the septum, anterior and lateral walls of the LV. The shorter, thicker left posterior fascicle supplies the electrical impulse to the posterior wall of the LV. A network of Purkinje fibres deliver the impulse first to the papillary muscles and then rapidly across the ventricles, resulting in simultaneous contraction. If the SA node fails to fire, the AV node, His-Purkinje system and ventricular myocardium are capable of generating an electrical impulse but at a slower rate than the SA node.

Movement of ions across the cell membrane, using diffusion and active transport mechanisms, is necessary to initiate myocardial depolarisation (systole) and repolarisation (diastolic relaxation).

The movement of ions across the cell membrane, known as the cardiac action potential, is responsible for initiating myocardial depolarisation (systole) and repolarisation (relaxation). A difference in electrical charge exists across the cell membrane, created by differences in the concentration of ions in the intracellular and extracellular fluid. This is known as the transmembrane potential. During the resting phase of the cardiac cycle, the transmembrane potential is approximately −90 mV (phase 4). At this stage, there is a higher concentration of intracellular potassium and lower concentration of intracellular sodium relative to their respective extracellular levels. This creates a concentration gradient, permitting the movement of ions across the cell membrane by diffusion and altering the transmembrane potential. Once this reaches −70 mV (threshold potential), early myocardial depolarisation will be triggered. Therefore, a sodium-potassium (Na^+/K^+) pump within the cell membrane uses active transport to move sodium out of the cell and potassium back into the cell to maintain the resting transmembrane potential of −90 mV during phase 4.

Myocardial depolarisation begins when sodium channels within the cell membrane open, permitting entry of sodium into the cell (phase 0). Once the transmembrane potential reaches the threshold potential of approximately −70 mV, fast sodium channels open, increasing the transmembrane potential to +30 mV. Repolarisation of the cell begins immediately afterwards, with a slight drop in transmembrane potential due to the closure of the sodium channels and an influx of chloride ions (phase 1). Myocardial contraction is maintained through the influx of calcium ions into the cell, causing the transmembrane potential to plateau at approximately 0 mV (phase 2). Repolarisation continues as the potassium channels open, allowing potassium to leave the cell, causing a dramatic fall in transmembrane potential (phase 3) until the resting membrane potential of −90 mV is reached and maintained using the Na^+/K^+ pump, rendering the cell inactive again (phase 4).

Coronary circulation

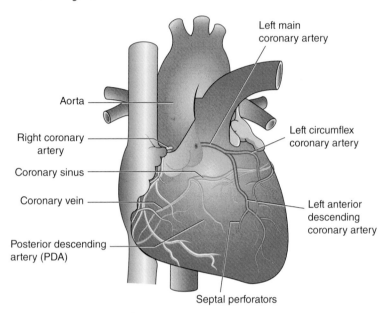

Left main
coronary artery

Aorta

Left circumflex
coronary artery

Right coronary
artery

Coronary sinus

Coronary vein

Left anterior
descending
coronary artery

Posterior descending
artery (PDA)

Septal perforators

Figure 1.3 Coronary circulation.

Situated within the epicardium, the coronary arterial circulation is
a network of arteries, arterioles and capillaries that penetrate the
myocardium to provide the oxygen and nutrients necessary for aerobic
metabolism (Figure 1.3). The right and left coronary arteries arise from
two sinuses positioned at the root of the aorta behind two of the aortic
valve cusps. Perfusion of the arteries occurs only during the diastolic
phase of the cardiac cycle as the cusps of the aortic valve obstruct the
sinuses during systole. The coronary arteries have four distinct layers of
tissue: the endothelium, tunica intima, media and adventitia.

The right coronary artery (RCA) extends along the right side of the
AV groove to the posterior wall of the heart, from where it proceeds
inferiorly towards the apex and then terminates. The RCA provides
perfusion for the right atrium, RV and the inferior surface of the LV,
as well as the SA and AV node, in the majority of the population. The
RCA also perfuses the posterior fascicle of the left bundle branch via
the posterior descending artery (PDA).

The left coronary artery emerges from the aortic root, extending
down the left atrium to the AV groove, where it bifurcates into the left
anterior descending (LAD) and circumflex arteries. The LAD gives rise
to diagonal branches and septal perforators, which perfuse the
anterior surface of the LV, the anterior papillary muscle and the
anterior aspect of the interventricular septum, including the right

bundle branch and the left anterior fascicle of the left bundle branch. The circumflex extends around the left AV groove to supply the lateral wall of the LV, via the obtuse marginal branches, as well as the left posterior fascicle, which is also supplied by the LAD.

The term dominance is used to describe the RCA when it perfuses the PDA, supplying the posterior wall of the LV and the AV nodal artery. Approximately 80–85% of the population have a dominant RCA. The circumflex is considered the dominant vessel in approximately 10–15% of the population, when the PDA emerges from the circumflex. A co-dominant circulation exists in approximately 5% of people in which both the RCA and circumflex extend to supply the posterior wall of the LV.

A collateral circulation exists between arterioles across the myocardium. In addition, portions of the subendocardial layer of myocardium may be perfused directly from the LV via the Thebesian veins.

Venous return from the myocardium occurs via the coronary veins, which follow the same route as the arterial circulation. The coronary veins drain into the coronary sinus, a large vessel situated along the posterior AV groove, which returns the deoxygenated blood into the right atrium. The myocardium also has a lymphatic circulation, which is also aligned with the arterial circulation.

Part 2 Rapid Cardiac Assessment

Rapid Cardiac Care, First Edition. Emma Menzies-Gow and Christine Spiers.
© 2018 John Wiley & Sons Ltd. Published 2018 by John Wiley & Sons Ltd.

Introduction

A systematic approach to patient assessment is fundamental to undertaking a comprehensive review of the acutely ill adult. The assessment should raise concerns about red flags, identify unsuspected problems and generate logical differential diagnosis to guide investigation and treatment. A set of vital signs: respiratory rate and character, oxygen saturations, heart rate and rhythm, bilateral blood pressure (BP), temperature and blood glucose will allow comparison of patient findings to those expected in a normal subject.

Cardiac history taking

The history-taking process is fundamental and should not be omitted unless the patient is in a critical state and requires an ABDCE assessment. Accurate history taking should take a systematic approach and be conducted in a logical manner.

Presenting complaint

A variety of cardiac and non-cardiac specific symptoms may be elicited; cardinal symptoms include:

- Chest/arm/back pain – tightness or discomfort.
- Breathlessness – on exertion, lying flat, at night.
- Palpitations – fast, slow, irregular.
- Syncope/fainting/dizziness – related to exercise, on standing, at rest.
- Pain in legs or calves – on walking, at rest.
- Ankle swelling.

Symptom assessment

Further elucidation of the symptom/complaint should establish the frequency, duration, exacerbation and severity of symptoms; assessment tools provide a framework for assessment and SOCRATES is a popular tool:

S – Site
O – Onset
C – Character
R – Radiation
A – Associated symptoms
T – Timing
E – Exacerbating factors
S – Severity.

Chest pain assessment

Chest pain is a commonly presenting symptom and the underlying diagnosis may range from trivial to potentially life threatening. Assessment can be augmented with the addition of other tests such as 12-lead ECG, blood tests for markers of cardiac injury (Troponin, CK-MB) or infection (CRP). Echocardiography, CXR and CT scans can provide further valid information. Cardiac causes of chest pain include acute coronary syndromes (ACS), pericarditis, myocarditis and aortic dissection. Respiratory conditions such as pneumonia, pneumothorax and pulmonary embolism can also present with chest pain. Musculoskeletal causes of chest pain include chest wall injuries, costochondritis and secondary tumours of the ribs.

> **S - Site** – the pain of myocardial ischaemia may be located in the jaw, throat, both arms, retrosternally and in the back. The pain from

pericarditis may be in the central chest, back or in the shoulders. Aortic dissection pain is located retrosternally and radiates into the back and the abdomen.

O - Onset – angina may be precipitated by exercise, emotion or cold weather. Pain associated with ACS may present at rest, on exertion or in the early hours of the morning on wakening. Pericardial pain may follow a period of flu-like symptoms or occur 3-6 weeks after acute MI.

C - Character – myocardial ischaemia is described as tight and crushing, but may also be an ache or heaviness. Aortic dissection pain has a tearing quality and pericardial pain is severe and constant.

R - Radiation – cardiac pain tends to radiate; ischaemic pain may radiate from the chest to the arms, jaw or back. The pain of aortic dissection often radiates into the back and occasionally the abdomen. Pericardial pain is frequently referred to the trapezius ridge (shoulder).

A - Associated symptoms – patients with myocardial infarction may present with dyspnoea, diaphoresis, nausea, syncope and extreme anxiety. Patients with ACS may present with one or several symptoms. In pericarditis, the pain is worse on inspiration. Aortic dissection may be associated with collapse and neurological involvement if a major vessel to the head and neck is compromised by the dissection.

T - Timing – myocardial ischaemia may have a sudden onset and the pain may last for longer than 20 minutes without relief. Aortic dissection tends to be of sudden onset and remains constant. Pericarditis and myocarditis may be preceded by a history of viral or flu-like symptoms.

E - Exacerbating factors – angina may be exacerbated by exercise, emotion, following meals or extreme weather temperatures. Pericardial pain is relieved by leaning forwards and made worse by deep inspiration.

S - Severity – whilst many patients with cardiac pain will describe the pain on the high end of a scale of 0–10, some patients, notably older patients and those with diabetes may experience little or no pain.

Risk factors

An evaluation of lifestyle and risk factors pertinent to cardiac disease should be undertaken. It is important to be non-judgemental but to ask questions sensitively and objectively. Key lifestyle factors include: cigarette smoking, misuse of alcohol, recreational drug use, lack of exercise and/or obesity. Cigarette smoking is the strongest modifiable risk factor for heart disease. Seek to evaluate if the patient has ever smoked and if so, how much and for how many years. Clarification of number of pack years is calculated by the following formula and is used to estimate the risk of smoking-related health problems:

$$\frac{\text{Number of cigarettes smoked per day} \times \text{Number of years smoked}}{20 \text{ (number of cigarettes per pack)}}$$

Estimate the amount of alcohol consumed per week; hazardous drinking is more than 2 units of alcohol per day for women, 3 units for men. One unit of alcohol is equivalent to a small glass of wine or half a pint of beer. Excessive alcohol use is implicated in hypertension, atrial fibrillation and dilated cardiomyopathy.

The increasing use of recreational drugs, particularly amphetamines and 'legal highs', is implicated in tachyarrhythmias. Cocaine may cause coronary artery vasospasm leading to ACS. Intravenous drug injection may act as a source for bacterial endocarditis. Obesity increases the risk of heart disease by inducing hypertension, hyperlipidaemia and diabetes. Diabetes is a significant risk factor for vascular and heart disease. Diabetes also magnifies the effects of other risk factors for cardiovascular disease.

Medications and allergies

Establish whether any medications have been prescribed and question whether these are being taken. The patient's current medications may help to confirm a suspected diagnosis, whilst newly prescribed drugs may have caused or aggravated symptoms; bronchodilators may precipitate tachycardia, beta-blockers may exacerbate heart failure or peripheral vascular disease and calcium channel blockers can cause oedema. Specific questioning around alternative, supplementary or 'over-the-counter' medications may raise suspicion of a drug-induced event; 'recreational' drugs such as cocaine may induce coronary artery spasm and ACS. Take note of any known allergies to medications.

Family history

Any known inherited or familial problems should be documented. A positive family history is a specific risk factor in coronary heart disease, and premature death in first degree relatives (<55 in males, < 60 years in females) indicates a familial risk. Similarly, a sudden premature death in the family may indicate undiagnosed arrhythmic syndromes such as Brugada or Long QT syndrome or structural abnormalities such as Hypertrophic Cardiomyopathy. Familial hyperlipidaemia leads to premature coronary artery disease and familial clotting disorders may precipitate venous thromboembolism.

Past medical history (PMH)

PMH and cardiovascular risk factors should be considered in the context of the presenting complaint. Links between other diseases such as hypertension, diabetes mellitus, respiratory and renal disease should also be considered. Recent cytotoxic therapy may be the aetiology of acute heart failure, whereas obstructive pulmonary disease may lead to chronic right-sided heart failure. Hyperthyroidism may cause tachyarrhythmias such as atrial fibrillation and patients with Marfan's syndrome may present with acute aortic dissection. Immunisation and any recent foreign travel may also be relevant.

Physical examination

The aim of the physical examination is to gather objective data to confirm or refute any differential diagnoses identified from the focussed history. Initial assessment should clarify if the patient is in pain or anxious, and any evidence of dyspnoea, pallor, diaphoresis or cyanosis would require urgent investigation. Examination of the cardiovascular system should include the whole circulatory system, not just the heart and utilises the following approach: inspection, palpation and auscultation.

Inspection

Inspection of the face, eyes, neck, hands, feet and chest will often provide evidence of heart disease. Facial dysmorphic features raise the suspicion of Down's syndrome and William's syndrome, which may cause significant structural heart disease. Evidence of hyperlipidaemia may be evident in xanthelasma (yellowish deposits in the skin near the eyelids) or corneal arcus (a white ring around the iris). Malar flush may be associated with mitral stenosis or chronic low-output states. Pallor may indicate anaemia (a cause of chest pain), and cyanosis is seen in patients with cyanotic congenital heart disease. Pallor and cyanosis is best evaluated in the mucous membranes of the eyes or by inspection of the mouth and tongue. Gingivitis and poor dental hygiene is a common source of bacterial endocarditis. A high arched palate with crowded teeth is seen in patients with Marfan syndrome.

Evaluate the neck for evidence of jugular venous distension (JVD), which is seen in right-sided heart failure, pericardial constriction or superior vena cava obstruction. Raised JVD is identified if the jugular pulsation can be seen more than 3 cm above the clavicle with reference to the sternal notch when a patient is lying at an angle of 45°. The hands are a good source of cardiac signs – clubbing of the fingers is seen in cyanotic congenital heart disease, peripheral cyanosis may be evident at the fingertips and splinter haemorrhages may be evident in bacterial endocarditis. Chest wall or sternal abnormalities, such as pectus excavatum (funnel chest) or pectus carinatum (pigeon chest), may displace the heart and limit cardiac function. Any evidence of previous cardiac surgery (sternotomy or chest drain scars) and any infraclavicular scars from placement of cardiac devices (pacemakers and implantable cardioverter defibrillators) should be noted. Evaluation of the legs and feet for oedema, skin discolouration or loss of hair growth may indicate heart failure, peripheral vascular disease or venous insufficiency.

Palpation

Evaluate the rate, rhythm, character and volume of the peripheral pulses. Absence of a pulse is often indicative of ischaemia due to atherosclerosis or embolism. The radial pulse should be 60–100 beats per minute (bpm) in an adult. Bradycardia (heart rate less than 60 bpm) may be normal in athletes and during sleep, but may also indicate hypothyroidism, heart block (AV block) or be drug induced – (Digoxin or beta-blockers). Tachycardia is normal during exercise or anxiety but may indicate sepsis, hyperthyroidism, shock due to blood or fluid loss, heart failure or drug overdose. Abnormalities of pulse volume or character are rare and generally seen when the underlying valvular disease such as aortic regurgitation and aortic stenosis is moderately severe. When a pulse is not palpable it may be audible by Doppler flow evaluation. Limb pulses should be equal and when deficits are identified this may be due to aortic dissection (radial to radial delay), aortic aneurysm (femoral to femoral delay), or atrial fibrillation (radial-apical deficit). The chest can be palpated for any evidence of palpable murmurs (thrills), heaves or thrusts in right ventricular or left ventricular enlargement. The apical impulse is identified in the fifth intercostal space in the mid-clavicular line and deviation from this site may indicate left ventricular enlargement. A 'tapping' quality to the apex beat may be due to mitral stenosis, and a diffuse apical impulse is commonly associated with mitral regurgitation.

Auscultation

The auscultation landmarks are identified in Figure 2.1. These landmarks correspond to the place where the sounds generated by each heart valve is heard best. The sounds, referred to as 'lub-dup', relate to the closure of first the atrioventricular (tricuspid and mitral) followed by closure of the outlet (pulmonary and aortic) valves. The diaphragm of the stethoscope identifies high-pitched sounds (normal

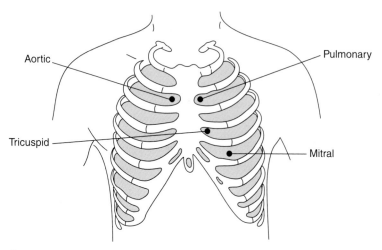

Figure 2.1 Cardiac auscultation landmarks.

heart sounds, systolic and diastolic murmurs), whereas the bell transmits the low-pitched sounds of mitral stenosis and the third and fourth heart sounds.

Auscultation of the lungs should include the anterior, posterior and lateral chest areas. Normal breath sounds are heard with the diaphragm of the stethoscope and include bronchial, broncho-vesicular and vesicular sounds.

Commonly identified murmurs in acute cardiac care include: third heart sound heard in heart failure, ejection systolic murmur in aortic stenosis and pan-systolic murmur in mitral regurgitation. Adventitious breath sounds in cardiac conditions include crackles associated with pulmonary oedema if bilateral and infection if unilateral.

Cardiac monitoring

Cardiac electrical activity can be recorded using a range of equipment that includes the 12-lead ECG and 3, 5 or 12-lead cardiac monitoring. Patients should be advised of the purpose of cardiac monitoring, their consent to proceed established and their dignity maintained throughout the procedure. The patient should be positioned comfortably and advised to remain resting while cardiac monitoring is being used, with a call bell available if help is needed. The electrodes must be placed directly onto clean, dry skin; hair may need to be removed to ensure good contact. If the patient's skin is clammy or has been recently moisturised, their skin should be cleaned with soap and water and thoroughly dried before applying electrodes.

In 3-lead monitoring, the limb lead electrodes should be positioned equidistant from the patient's heart around the upper chest and lower abdomen or on the upper and lower limbs, in the following sequence: Right Arm (red), Left Arm (yellow), Left Leg (green/black). If a fourth lead is available, this should be placed on the Right Leg (black). 5-lead monitoring involves an additional white lead, which should be connected to an electrode placed in the V_1 position (Figure 2.2). If 12-lead ECG monitoring is available, the electrodes should be positioned as for the 12-lead ECG.

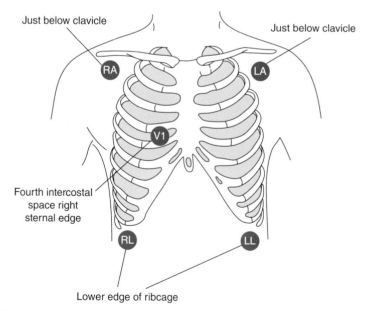

Figure 2.2 5-lead cardiac monitoring.

Lead II should be selected as it provides the clearest view of both atrial and ventricular activity. The size of the trace on the screen should be adjusted to ensure all waveforms are clearly visible. Artefact, or electrical interference, can severely affect the quality of the recording and impede rhythm recognition. It can be minimised by advising the patient to avoid excessive movement, ensuring the electrodes have good contact with skin and by limiting interference from nearby electrical equipment. The monitor alarm parameters should be adjusted for individual patients to alert the healthcare professional of a rise or fall in heart rate that may indicate the need for further assessment.

Rapid rhythm recognition

Once cardiac monitoring using lead II is established, systematic assessment can facilitate rapid rhythm recognition:

Assess ventricular rate and rhythm
Assess the QRS duration
Assess atrial activity, rate and rhythm
Assess relationship between atrial and ventricular activity
Assess PR and QT intervals
Identify the rhythm

The monitor records heart rate accurately but it can also be calculated from an ECG rhythm strip using the following formula:

$$\text{Heart rate} = \frac{1500}{\text{the number of small squares between two QRS complexes}}$$

Sinus rhythm: Normal waveforms and intervals

Sinus rhythm is the normal heart rhythm originating from the sino-atrial node. It is present when sequential conduction of the atria and ventricles, as described in Part 1, generates P, QRS and T waveforms that emerge from an isoelectric line. It is a regular rhythm, identified when the interval between consecutive QRS complexes, known as the R-R interval, is regular and constant, with a rate of between 60 and 100 bpm (Figure 2.3).

Normal atrial depolarisation, originating from the sinoatrial node, creates a small rounded P wave that emerges from the isoelectric line. In sinus rhythm, the P wave will be positive in lead II, appearing before the QRS complex. Each P wave should be followed by a QRS complex and T wave, representing ventricular depolarisation and repolarisation. The QRS duration will be less than 100 ms, indicating normal ventricular depolarisation using the His-Purkinje system. T waves should follow the direction of the QRS complex (concordant) in lead II, but can only be fully assessed using the 12-lead ECG.

The PR interval is a measurement taken to evaluate the delay in transmission though the AV node. Normally, the PR interval is 120–200 ms, measured from the beginning of the P wave to the beginning of the QRS complex. The QT interval is a measurement of the time taken for ventricular depolarisation and repolarisation to occur, measured from the beginning of the QRS complex to the end of the T wave. Rapid identification of a normal QT interval can be established if the QT interval is less than half the preceding R-R interval. However, as the QT interval is inversely proportional to rate, the corrected QT (QTc) interval should be calculated using Bazett's formula: $QT/\sqrt{RR}$ interval, as it adjusts the interval correctly for variation in heart rate.

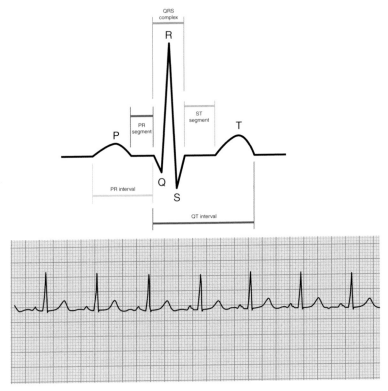

Figure 2.3 Normal ECG waveforms and sinus rhythm (lead II).

Sinus tachycardia

Sinus tachycardia is present when sinus rhythm has a QRS rate greater than 100 bpm. Stress and anxiety may cause an increase in sympathetic activity, increasing the sinoatrial node firing rate. However, sinus tachycardia may also occur in response to pain, ACS, sepsis, shock, heart failure or use of recreational drugs.

Sinus bradycardia

Sinus bradycardia is present when the sinus rhythm has a QRS rate of less than 60 bpm. This may be associated with high levels of fitness but may also be due to hypoxia, myocardial ischaemia, hypothermia or drugs that interfere with nodal conduction, such as beta-blockers.

Sinus arrhythmia

Sinus rhythm may appear to be irregular in some patients, particularly young people and the very elderly. This is known as sinus arrhythmia but is not considered an abnormal finding.

Cardiac investigations
Blood tests

A range of venous blood tests can provide data to aid the assessment, diagnosis and management of patients with suspected cardiac disease. Measurement of serum troponin I or T is useful in the diagnosis of patients presenting with chest pain or other symptoms associated with ACS. Troponin is a protein released as a result of myocardial damage. Most assays will begin to detect troponin around 4–6 hours after symptom onset. The sensitivity of available assays is improving with the emergence of high sensitivity troponins, able to detect troponin rise within 0–3 hours in patients with suspected ACS. However, other conditions may elevate troponin levels, such as arrhythmias, heart failure and chronic kidney disease. Creatine kinase (CK) and an isoenzyme of CK, CK-MB, are supplemental biochemical markers of current myocardial damage.

Elevated or low levels of potassium, magnesium, sodium, and calcium levels may cause atrial or ventricular ectopic beats and arrhythmias. Urea, creatinine levels and estimated glomerular filtration rate (eGFR) are used to assess renal function, which may be impaired in patients with cardiac conditions such as heart failure. Evaluation of renal function is particularly important for patients prior to coronary angiography or primary percutaneous coronary intervention (P-PCI), due to administration of radio-opaque contrast. The contrast is excreted by the kidneys and thus must be used with caution in patients with renal dysfunction.

The BNP and NT-pro-BNP will be elevated in patients with left ventricular dysfunction. Both assays correlate with the severity of heart failure and are predictive of cardiovascular events and mortality.

Liver function tests, including AST, ALT, LDH and ALP, may indicate hepatic dysfunction associated with heart failure or reveal a coagulopathy. Hyperthyroidism and hypothyroidism are both known risk factors for cardiovascular disease. Capillary blood glucose, fasting glucose and HbA1c assays are useful to diagnose diabetes, a known risk factor for cardiovascular disease and to ascertain the presence of hyperglycaemia during ACS. A fasting lipid profile can be used to guide lifestyle advice and medical therapy for patients with hyperlipidaemia. A full blood count will provide evidence of anaemia or infection.

Arterial and venous blood gases provide information on oxygen and carbon dioxide levels, acid-base balance and lactate levels, providing useful data in patients with, for example, dyspnoea and sepsis.

The 12-lead electrocardiograph (ECG)

A 12-lead ECG can be used to identify myocardial ischaemia and arrhythmia. Patients with symptoms of chest, neck, arm, jaw or abdominal pain should have a 12-lead ECG as this may reveal ischaemia, as should patients presenting with palpitations, dyspnoea and syncopal symptoms. Ambulatory 24-hour ECG (Holter) monitoring and event recording can be used to identify paroxysmal arrhythmias, to record heart rate variability or a signal-averaged ECG, and to guide the use of implantable cardioverter defibrillator (ICDs). Tilt testing, during which BP and an ECG are continuously recorded, may be used to investigate patients with syncopal symptoms or vasovagal episodes. The ECG may used in exercise tolerance testing, in which the patient walks or runs on a treadmill to ascertain the presence of arrhythmia or ischaemia, although the use of this test is diminishing with the emergence of more sensitive imaging techniques such as stress echocardiography.

Cardiac imaging

The cardiac structures can be visualised using a chest X-ray taken in the posterior-anterior (PA) view and, if required, the lateral view when the patient has taken a deep breath. Chest X-ray (CXR) can facilitate assessment of heart size, dimensions of the thoracic aorta and pulmonary artery and signs of pericardial effusion, atrial and ventricular enlargement and ascending aortic dissection. A CXR may reveal signs of pulmonary oedema associated with heart failure.

Echocardiography uses ultrasound to assess cardiac function. A trans-thoracic echocardiogram (TTE) is recorded by placing a transducer on the patient's chest while they are lying on their left side, with their left arm out. A TTE can examine the movement of the chambers, septum and valves and approximate left ventricular ejection fraction, normally 50–65%. Doppler can be used to ascertain direction of blood flow, valuable in diagnosing valvular regurgitation. Three-dimensional echocardiography can be used to aid diagnosis of mitral and aortic disease and congenital heart disease. Stress echocardiography can establish the presence of hibernating or stunned myocardium. The 'stress' is produced through administration of dobutamine or by conducting the scan while the patient walks or runs on a treadmill, although there is an associated risk of inducing ventricular arrhythmias. Transoesophageal echocardiography (TOE), in which the transducer is advanced into the oesophagus, can provide high-quality images of valvular function and is used to visualise vegetation associated with endocarditis. This procedure requires local anaesthesia and sedation and is frequently used in the intensive care setting.

Cardiac magnetic resonance (CMR) imaging is an increasingly popular non-invasive technique used to investigate patients with cardiovascular disease. CMR can be used to provide diagnostic information for patients with a variety of cardiac conditions including ischaemic, aortic, congenital and valvular heart disease. It is a non-invasive procedure that does not expose the patient to radiation nor require anaesthesia or sedation but may be unsuitable for patients with certain cardiac devices such as pacemakers.

A computed tomography (CT) coronary angiogram, using a peripheral infusion of contrast, is highly effective in the diagnosis of coronary artery disease. Other non-invasive cardiac investigations include the use of CT scans to assess the thoracic aorta if aneurysm or dissection is suspected and to undertake coronary artery calcium scoring in patients with ischaemic heart disease. A 'thallium' scan is a nuclear imaging test during which radioactive thallium is administered intravenously to identify areas of viable myocardium that may respond to reperfusion with coronary bypass graft surgery.

Invasive cardiac investigations

Cardiac catheterisation is an invasive procedure used to conduct coronary angiograms, aortography and investigate right heart function. During a coronary angiogram, X-rays are recorded of coronary blood flow while radio-opaque dye is injected into the right and left coronary arteries via a catheter inserted into the right femoral or radial artery. It can also be used to assess left ventricular ejection fraction. Angiography can be used to diagnose ischaemic heart disease and to determine if the patient would benefit from insertion of an intracoronary stent or from coronary artery bypass graft surgery.

Right heart function can be assessed using a venous catheter advanced into the right ventricle and pulmonary artery to directly measure pressure within each chamber. Pulmonary arterial 'wedge' pressure can be used as an indirect measure of left atrial pressure and left ventricular end-diastolic pressure. This test is conducted in patients prior to cardiac transplantation and in those with pulmonary hypertension.

In an electrophysiology study, electrodes are advanced via a venous catheter to locate abnormal electrical pathways, such as a re-entry circuit seen in supraventricular tachycardia (SVT). This information is used to establish the patient's suitability for interventions such as radiofrequency ablation, cryoablation or insertion of an ICD.

Part 3 Rapid 12-lead ECG Interpretation

Rapid Cardiac Care, First Edition. Emma Menzies-Gow and Christine Spiers.
© 2018 John Wiley & Sons Ltd. Published 2018 by John Wiley & Sons Ltd.

Introduction

The Electrocardiogram (ECG) is a graphic record of the electrical activity generated by the cells of the heart, recorded at the body surface by electrodes and displayed onto a cardiac monitor or ECG paper as a visual record. The electrodes detect the electrical current generated by depolarisation and repolarisation of the atria and ventricles during each cardiac cycle.

ECGs are recorded onto grid paper that records time in seconds along the horizontal axis, and voltage or amplitude in millivolts (mV) on the vertical axis. Each small square is equivalent to 1 mm or 40 ms in time and 5 small squares is separated by a dark vertical line representing 5 mm or 200 ms. The ECG should be calibrated and recorded at 25 mm/second and 1 mV should produce a 10 mm deflection on the ECG.

Whereas cardiac monitoring employs three or four leads monitoring in a single plane, a 12-lead ECG evaluates the heart in two planes utilising 12 leads or 'views' to evaluate the electrical activity. Four electrodes are applied to the limbs in the following sequence: Right Arm (red), Left Arm (yellow), Left Leg (green), Right Leg (black) and six electrodes are applied to the chest or precordium. These leads are referred to as the 'V' leads or 'chest' leads and are recorded by applying the electrodes to prescribed areas over the anterior chest wall (V_1–V_6).

Simply put, an ECG lead is a recording of the heart's electrical activity from one viewpoint, the 12-lead ECG views the heart from 12 perspectives and helps to build up a three-dimensional picture of the cardiac electrical activity. Six of the leads view the frontal plane of the body and these leads are derived from the four electrodes placed on the limbs (the 'limb leads'). Leads V_1–V_6 view the horizontal or transverse plane of the body and are referred to as the 'chest leads' (Figure 3.1).

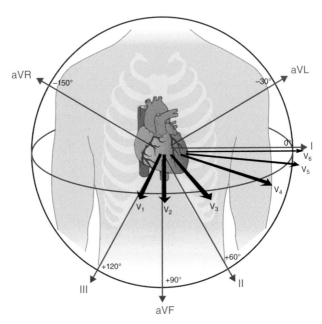

Figure 3.1 Orientation of the 12 ECG leads.

Cardiac vectors and axis

Atrial and ventricular depolarisation and repolarisation generates an electrical current that flows from the sino-atrial node, towards the atrio-ventricular node and downwards through the His-Purkinje system towards the left ventricular apex. The electrical current is described as the cardiac vector or the cardiac axis and this is a composite view of the general direction of the electrical current (Figure 3.2). The average direction of the vectors that result from ventricular depolarisation is called the mean QRS axis and this can be calculated using the 360° circle known as the hexaxial reference figure on which are inscribed the six limb leads. The figure is divided into quadrants by the bisection of lead axis I (at 0° on the circle) and aVF (at +90° on the circle). Axis deviation can result from many cardiac abnormalities and its calculation is an essential part of the initial interpretation of the 12-lead ECG.

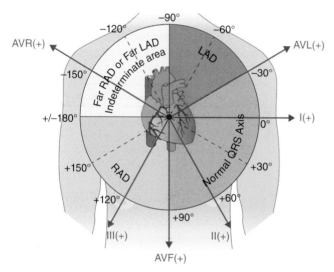

Figure 3.2 Hexaxial reference system showing four quadrants – normal, left, right and indeterminate axis.

Rapid ECG analysis tool

Rapid ECG assessment in the cardiac patient utilises a quick and systematic tool, which ensures that significant abnormalities are identified early and that important information is not missed.

Significant QRS abnormalities (QRS confounders) should be identified early: Wolff-Parkinson-White (WPW), bundle branch block (BBB) and fascicular block, all of which cause electrical impulses to be conducted abnormally throughout the ventricles and may mimic ischaemia and infarction to complicate the diagnosis. In this tool, significant QRS confounders are ruled out first before looking for evidence of myocardial ischaemia or infarction:

Rapid ECG Analysis Assessment:

Heart rate and rhythm using the rhythm analysis tool
QRS axis
Evidence of pre-excitation
Evidence of bundle branch and fascicular blocks
Evidence of myocardial ischaemia and infarction
Evidence of other conditions guided by the patient's clinical presentation

---

Rate and rhythm assessment

Heart rate and cardiac rhythm is an important aspect of patient assessment and this should be evaluated first by the analysis tool.

Assess ventricular rate and rhythm
Assess the QRS duration
Assess atrial activity, rate and rhythm
Assess relationship between atrial and ventricular activity
Assess PR and QT intervals
Identify the rhythm

QRS axis calculation

The QRS axis reflects the general direction of the electrical current as it flows across the heart. Normally the QRS axis is directed downwards and to the left due to the dominance of the left ventricle. The QRS axis is identified by using the hexaxial reference system and is measured using the frontal plane leads. A simple three-step method facilitates the measurement of the mean frontal plane QRS axis and is based on the understanding that the biphasic lead is 90° to the mean frontal plane axis. This method of axis determination is quick, simple and accurate:

1. Identify the biphasic lead – this is the lead which has the most equal positive and negative components and is often the smallest QRS complex.
2. Identify the lead that is oriented 90° or perpendicular to this lead using the hexaxial reference system.
3. Consider the direction of the QRS complex in the lead identified in step 2. If the QRS is predominantly positive, the axis is heading towards this lead on the hexaxial reference system. If the QRS is predominantly negative, the axis is heading away from this lead (identified as the negative pole on the hexaxial reference system). A list of possible causes of axis deviation is provided in Table 3.1.

Table 3.1 Causes of axis deviation

Right axis deviation +90° to +180°	Left axis deviation −30° to −90°
Can be normal in thin, tall, young individuals	Can be normal in elderly patients, obesity and third trimester of pregnancy
RBBB	LBBB
RVH	LVH
Left posterior fascicular block	Left anterior fascicular block
Pre-excitation syndrome left sided accessory pathway	Pre-excitation right-sided accessory pathway
Lateral wall myocardial infarction	Inferior wall myocardial infarction
COPD or acute pulmonary embolism	Hyperkalaemia
Dextracardia	Artificial cardiac pacing

Pre-excitation syndromes

The characteristic findings of shortened PR interval (<120 ms), a delta wave (a slurring of the proximal portion of the QRS) altering the normal shape, duration and voltage of the QRS complex and a subsequent discordant ST segment or T wave is the characteristic ECG pattern of ventricular pre-excitation known as Wolff-Parkinson-White (WPW) (Figure 3.3). Both WPW and a rarer form of ventricular pre-excitation, which results in a short PR interval but no other significant ECG abnormalities, put the patient at risk of supraventricular tachycardia.

The presence of accessory pathways, which conduct electrical impulses from the atria to the ventricles, bypassing the atrio-ventricular (AV) node, produces these characteristic ECG findings. This notching and widening of the QRS complex with discordant ST segments and T waves can mimic other pathological conditions including BBB, ventricular hypertrophy and myocardial infarction and therefore ventricular pre-excitation must be ruled out early in the ECG analysis. The accessory pathways may bypass the AV node with subsequent loss of the protective decremental properties of the AV node and allows a potentially fatal tachyarrhythmia to evolve.

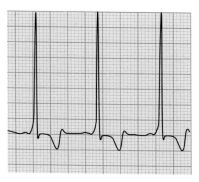

Figure 3.3 WPW pattern.

Bundle branch block and fascicular block

Bundle branch block and fascicular block typically cause axis deviation and abnormalities of the QRS complexes, ST-segments and T waves.

The intraventricular conduction system rapidly conducts electrical impulses to the ventricles. The right bundle branch (RBB) carries impulses to the right ventricle, and the left anterior fascicle and left posterior fascicle of the left bundle branch (LBB) depolarise the left ventricle. Normal conduction to the ventricles is fast and depolarisation of the ventricles occurs in a right to left sequence producing characteristic QRS complexes which are narrow (<100 ms). The initial depolarisation of the interventricular septum by the LBB is from left to right producing a small 'septal' r wave in V_1 lead. This is followed by simultaneous depolarisation of the right and left ventricles with the mean direction of current from right to left and thus the QRS complex primarily reflects depolarisation of the left ventricle.

When BBB occurs, the ventricle affected depolarises slower and aberrantly producing: QRS > 100 ms, abnormal QRS complexes with notching, ST segment and T wave abnormalities and axis deviation. The findings of BBB are best evaluated in the chest leads, primarily in V_1 and V_6.

Right Bundle Branch Block (RBBB)

A typical RBBB pattern produces a wide QRS complex (>100 ms) with an rSR' wave in V_1 and V_2 (Figure 3.4) and a slurred S wave in V_6, with possible right axis deviation and ST and T wave abnormalities seen in V_1 and V_2.

In RBBB, septal activation occurs in the normal way from the LBB, and this wave of current is from left to right resulting in the normal small 'r' wave in V_1. The left ventricle is activated through the normally functioning LBB, causing an S wave in V_1 as the impulses travel away from the V_1 lead. The right ventricle depolarises late and abnormally via the myocardial cell structure, causing delayed RV activation and this results in a wide second R wave in V_1, V_2 (the characteristic rSR' pattern) and a slurred S wave in V_6. There may also be right axis deviation and ST and T wave abnormalities in the right-sided chest leads.

Left Bundle Branch Block (LBBB)

The left ventricle and the left bundle branch dominate the electrical forces on the ECG and thus LBBB produces changes, which are manifest in *most* or *all* leads on the 12-lead ECG. LBBB produces wide notched QRS complexes (>100 ms) in all ECG leads, QS (negative QRS) or rS in V_1 (Figure 3.5), a broad positive QRS in V_5, V_6, ST-segment deviation and T wave discordancy in *all* ECG leads. In particular, the

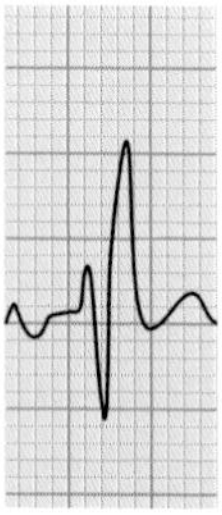

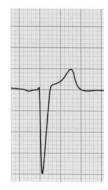

Figure 3.4 rSR' pattern associated with RBBB as seen in V$_1$.

Figure 3.5 QS pattern associated with LBBB as seen in V$_1$.

patient may exhibit ST-segment elevation in V$_1$–V$_3$, which can mimic MI to the untrained eye.

In LBBB, the septum does not depolarise in the normal left to right direction and this causes the loss of the 'septal r wave' in V$_1$. The left ventricle depolarises late and abnormally via cell-to-cell conduction and this produces a wide (and sometimes notched) QRS complex in all leads. Additionally, there is abnormal repolarisation of the myocardial tissue and this results in ST segment and T wave discordance seen in all ECG leads.

Fascicular block

Fascicular block refers to abnormal, delayed or blocked conduction through the left anterior or left posterior fascicle of the LBB. Abnormal conduction through these fascicles disrupts normal ventricular depolarisation producing characteristic changes to QRS morphology and axis deviation.

Left anterior fascicular block (LAFB) causes left axis deviation of greater than −45° with an rS pattern in aVF and III, qR pattern in I and aVL.

Left posterior block causes right axis deviation of greater than 120° with a qR pattern in aVF and III and rS in I and aVL.

LAFB is more common than left posterior fascicular block, as the left anterior fascicle is more vulnerable to damage because of its anatomic position, single blood supply and close association with the aortic valve.

Bifascicular block

Fascicular blocks can occur alone or in conjunction with RBBB. LAFB and RBBB is the more usual presentation of bifascicular block (due to the shared LAD blood supply). Bifascicular block may deteriorate into complete heart block, particularly in the presence of acute MI. In the presence of first-degree AV block, trifascicular block is said to be present.

Myocardial ischaemia or infarction

Acute coronary syndromes (ACS) are sudden life-threatening events, which demonstrate classic ECG changes that are sequential and dynamic and create changes in T waves, ST segments and the Q wave:

- Myocardial ischaemia – T wave changes and ST-segment deviation.
- Myocardial infarction – ST-segment deviation and Q waves.

12-lead ECG changes indicative of ST-segment elevation myocardial infarction (STEMI) are:

- ST-segment elevation > 1 mm in any two contiguous leads except for V_2 and V_3 where the following rules apply:
  - Males under 40 years ST-segment elevation > 2.5 mm.
  - Males over 40 years ST-segment elevation > 2 mm.
  - Females any age ST-segment elevation > 1.5 mm.

12-lead ECG changes indicative of non-STEMI or unstable angina are:

- ST-segment depression 0.5 mm in two contiguous leads.
- T wave inversion in two contiguous leads.

Myocardial infarction and ischaemia manifest changes in the ST segments and T waves as indicated in Figures 3.6a–c.

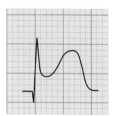

Figure 3.6a ST elevation.

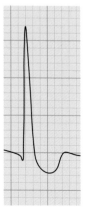

Figure 3.6b ST depression.

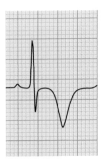

Figure 3.6c T wave inversion.

The leads in which these changes occur reflect the anatomical location of the damage, the likely culprit coronary artery and potential complications that can be identified in the Table 3.2 below:

Table 3.2 Possible complications due to 12-lead ECG changes

Culprit coronary artery	Anatomical territory/infarct area	ECG leads	Possible complications
LAD (septal branch)	Antero-septal LV	V_1–V_2	RBBB, Bifascicular block, LVF
LAD (diagonal branch)	Anterior LV	V_3–V_4	RBBB, Bifascicular block, LVF
LCx	Anterolateral LV	V_5–V_6, 1 and aVL	LVF, AV block
LCx or RCA	Posterior LV	Tall R waves V_1, V_2 or leads V_7–V_9	LVF, AV block
RCA	Inferior LV	II, III, aVF	Sinus node arrhythmias and AV block
Proximal RCA	Right ventricle	V_3R and V_4R	Hypotension, right heart failure

LAD Left anterior descending; LCx Left circumflex; RCA right coronary artery

Consider specific conditions based on the patient's history and presentation

Chamber enlargement such as atrial or ventricular hypertrophy can produce ECG waves of increased amplitude, duration and axis deviation. Left ventricular hypertrophy is characterised by:

- Tall R waves in leads facing the LV – V_5, V_6, I and aVL.
- QRS axis $\leq -30°$.

- ST depression and/or T wave inversion in leads facing the LV – V_5, V_6, I and aVL.
- Wide notched P waves > 100 ms, demonstrating left atrial enlargement ('p mitrale').

Right ventricular hypertrophy is rare but is demonstrated by:

- Tall 'dominant' R waves in leads facing the RV – V_1 and V_2.
- QRS axis ≥ +90°.
- ST and/or T wave inversion in leads facing the RV – V_1 and V_2.
- Tall peaked P waves > 2.5 mm demonstrating right atrial enlargement ('p pulmonale').

Other clinical conditions may mimic the presence of infarction or make the ECG more difficult to analyse. Certain conditions such as Brugada syndrome, Takotsubo cardiomyopathy, arrhythmogenic right ventricular cardiomyopathy (ARVC), pericarditis and myocarditis can all produce ST-segment elevation on the ECG and these conditions are known as infarct imposters. The reader is advised to read the relevant chapters elsewhere in this book.

Other abnormalities seen on the 12-lead ECG

To conclude the analysis, the ECG findings should be considered in the context of the patient's presenting signs, symptoms and other clinical criteria. If the patient has clinical symptoms but the ECG remains normal, serial ECG recordings should be undertaken alongside other clinical examinations and assessments. Additionally, supplemental leads and serial ECG recordings should be made in patients with clinical symptoms of ischaemia but non-diagnostic ECGs. In patients with inferior and suspected right ventricular involvement, V_3R and V_4R may demonstrate ST-segment elevation. Posterior wall (infero-basal) infarction should be suspected in patients with tall R waves in V_1, V_2 and ST-segment depression and the addition of leads V_7–V_9 is strongly recommended to evaluate the posterior myocardial wall.

Part 4 Cardiac Conditions A–Z

Rapid Cardiac Care, First Edition. Emma Menzies-Gow and Christine Spiers.
© 2018 John Wiley & Sons Ltd. Published 2018 by John Wiley & Sons Ltd.

Acute coronary syndromes

'Acute coronary syndromes' (ACS) is an umbrella term referring to conditions caused by an episode of myocardial ischaemia occurring at rest or on minimal exertion. Sudden onset of chest pain is the most common symptom associated with ACS. The electrocardiogram (ECG) and cardiac biomarkers are used to differentiate between a diagnosis of ST-segment elevation myocardial infarction (STEMI), non-ST-segment elevation MI (NSTEMI) and unstable angina (UA). All three diagnoses are medical emergencies requiring rapid treatment to restore coronary perfusion and reduce the significant risk to mortality and morbidity.

Pathophysiology

ACS usually occur when there is erosion or disruption of a coronary atheromatous plaque, triggering thrombus formation within a coronary artery that can result in myocardial ischaemia, injury and necrosis (infarction). Cardiac risk factors such as hypertension, smoking and diabetes can contribute to the breakdown of the coronary endothelium and the fibrous cap around the plaque, leading to exposure of the thrombogenic lipid core to blood. This initiates rapid accumulation and activation of platelets and thrombosis within the coronary lumen. Activated platelets induce localised vasoconstriction, leading to rapid partial (NSTEMI/UA) or total occlusion (STEMI) of the coronary artery. This obstruction of coronary perfusion inhibits oxygenation of the myocardium beyond, causing ischaemia. Systolic activity of the ischaemic myocardium will initially continue while the myocytes function anaerobically. However, in the absence of rapid reperfusion, the affected portion of myocardium will soon cease contraction (myocardial injury) and eventually die (infarction).

History

Many patients live with chronic health issues that will significantly increase their risk of experiencing an ACS, such as diabetes, hypertension and obesity. Some have made lifestyle choices that also increase cardiovascular risk, such as smoking, adopting a high cholesterol, salt or sugar diet or taking limited or no regular exercise. Risk of ACS is significantly increased in patients who have a family history of heart disease and who may exhibit modifiable or non-modifiable risk factors that would contribute to the development of atherosclerosis.

Signs and symptoms

Many patients typically experience a sudden onset of retrosternal chest pain that is commonly described as a sharp pain, a crushing heaviness or a dull ache that radiates down their left arm or into their neck or lower jaw. These classic symptoms of ACS are caused by myocardial ischaemia. Others, particularly women, the elderly and patients with renal disease or diabetes, experience more ambiguous symptoms such as arm or jaw ache or heaviness, or nausea, vomiting and fatigue. Some will not experience any symptoms at all. The symptoms frequently commence at rest, for example while asleep, or during minimal exertion, but do not dissipate with rest or change in position. This differs significantly from the presentation of stable angina, where chest pain will ease with rest. Patients presenting with ACS may have had recent episodes of similar symptoms that have previously resolved, either with rest or with anti-anginal treatment, although for others this will be the first occurrence.

ACS can be life threatening and are the most common cause of sudden cardiac death among adults in the UK. Acute reduction in oxygenation of the myocardium not only induces chest pain but also increases the propensity for potentially fatal ventricular arrhythmias and acute heart failure, which could manifest as the initial clinical presentation. Additional symptoms may also be evident such as tachypnoea, arrhythmias, cool, clammy skin and a pale, grey pallor associated with increased sympathetic neurohormonal activity. Acute anxiety and distress frequently accompany ACS, with many patients expressing an overwhelming fear of imminent death. Ventricular tachycardia/ventricular fibrillation (VT/VF) cardiac arrest may occur soon after the onset of symptoms for which early defibrillation is essential to ensure survival.

The symptoms associated with ACS are common to all three diagnoses and, therefore, cannot be used to differentiate between UA, NSTEMI and STEMI. Similarly, the severity of symptoms is not a diagnostic indicator of the underlying form of ACS. Rapidly establishing a diagnosis is paramount for patients presenting with suspected ACS, to ensure that treatment is expedited swiftly to reduce the risk to mortality and long-term morbidity.

Assessment and investigations

Assessment should be prioritised to optimise patient safety. Initial observations should include assessment of respiratory rate, oxygen saturation level, pulse and blood pressure, which should be repeated at frequent intervals. Cardiac monitoring should be commenced rapidly to observe for arrhythmias and a 12-lead ECG recorded to diagnose or rule out ACS. If inconclusive, posterior and right ventricular lead ECGs should be recorded and the patient should have an urgent echocardiogram.

A focussed medical history should be obtained to ascertain the nature, onset and duration of the patient's symptoms and to establish the likelihood of ACS due to the existence of cardiac risk factors and family history of cardiac disease. Evaluating the nature, quality, onset and radiation of chest pain and the patient's response to anti-anginal therapy can be useful tools in establishing the likelihood of ACS where the ECG is inconclusive.

ACS is diagnosed from the patient's clinical presentation, ST-T wave changes on the 12-lead ECG and serum cardiac troponin levels. STEMI is present when there is 1 mm of ST-segment elevation, measured at the J point in two or more contiguous leads, other than in leads V_2 and V_3, where ST-segment elevation is higher and is age and gender specific. New left bundle branch block (LBBB) may also develop in the context of STEMI. The ECG changes associated with UA/NSTEMI are T wave inversion, ST-segment depression or transient ST-segment elevation in two contiguous leads. If the standard ECG is inconclusive, posterior (V_7–V_9) and right ventricular leads (V_3R and V_4R) should be recorded and analysed for signs of ischaemia.

A range of serum blood tests should be conducted, including samples for urea and electrolytes, cardiac troponins, full blood count and a clotting screen. Cardiac troponin levels should be assessed on initial presentation and repeated 12 hours later (high sensitivity troponin can be measured within 0 to 3 hours). The troponin level will be raised in STEMI and NSTEMI but remain negative in UA. GRACE and CRUSADE scores should be calculated to estimate prognosis and quantify bleeding risk respectively.

Treatment

Treatment of ACS should be expedited to ensure haemodynamic stability, alleviate symptoms and anxiety, establish coronary reperfusion and minimise short- and long-term risk of morbidity and mortality. Administration of opiate analgesia with anti-emetic should be prioritised while ensuring the patient remains on bed rest. Reassurance should be given where possible to help address anxiety. Resuscitation equipment should be immediately available, as patients with ACS are at risk of life-threatening arrhythmias and sudden cardiac death.

Dual anti-platelet (aspirin and P2Y12 inhibitor) and anti-thrombin therapies should be commenced as soon as possible in the absence of contraindications. Rapid delivery of primary percutaneous coronary intervention (P-PCI) is the mainstay of treatment for STEMI. Patients with NSTEMI/UA should also have percutaneous coronary intervention (PCI) but with less immediacy. However, PCI should be expedited for patients identified as being at high ischaemic risk by using the GRACE score or if the patient develops haemodynamic instability, refractory angina or life-threatening complications such as arrhythmias or heart failure.

Secondary prevention should be commenced at the earliest opportunity to prevent recurrence of ACS and complications associated with myocardial damage. Dual anti-platelet therapy should be continued in conjunction with a beta-blocker, an ACE-inhibitor and an HMG CoA reductase inhibitor (statin) in the absence of contraindications. Rivaroxaban may be commenced once the anti-thrombin agent has been stopped during the in-patient stay. Cardiac rehabilitation should be offered to patients 3–4 weeks post-discharge.

Acute coronary syndromes: treatment and interventions

Pathophysiology

Acute coronary syndromes (ACS) encompasses a range of clinical conditions which cause myocardial ischaemia, discussed in the preceding chapter. Patients who have sustained an ST-segment elevation myocardial infarction (STEMI) will undergo Primary Percutaneous Coronary Intervention (P-PCI) (angioplasty and stent implantation) but where timely P-PCI is not available, thrombolytic (fibrinolytic) therapy may be offered. Patients who have non-STEMI (NSTEMI) or unstable angina (UA) are also likely to undergo coronary angiography and intervention (stent deployment) to achieve perfusion to the jeopardised myocardium by reopening the culprit coronary artery. The onset of ACS generally results from rupture of the atheromatous plaque and exposure of the lipid core. Platelet adhesion at the site and platelet activation and aggregation leads to stimulation of the clotting cascade and potential thrombus formation. Antiplatelet therapy aims to inhibit platelet activation and aggregation and longer term pharmacological therapy aims to enhance thrombus resolution and prevent recurrent thrombotic events. In addition, optimisation of secondary preventive strategies prevents left ventricular remodelling and reduces the risk of further coronary events.

Antiplatelet strategies

Reducing platelet activation is crucial and, unless absolutely contraindicated, all patients should be prescribed *Aspirin* which exerts its antiplatelet effect by irreversibly binding to the cyclooxygenase-1 (COX-1) enzyme, reducing production of thromboxane A_2, a powerful vasoconstrictor. The addition of a second antiplatelet drug is indicated when a patient has received an intracoronary stent. Thienopyridines block the adenosine diphosphate (ADP) P2Y12 receptor on platelets and include *Clopidogrel*, *Prasugrel* and *Ticagrelor*. Clopidogrel is a prodrug that requires two stage metabolism to achieve the active metabolite. This results in a slow onset of efficacy and the dual hepatic activation results in variable individual patient response to the drug. The use of Prasugrel overcomes some of the limitations of Clopidogrel. Prasugrel also exerts its antiplatelet effect by irreversibly binding to the ADP P2Y12 receptor, but it only requires one metabolic step to become active and hence it achieves its effect faster and with less inter-patient variability of response. It does however cause an increased risk of bleeding and it is not recommended for use in patients older than 75 years or under 60 kg and patients who have previously sustained Transient Ischaemic Attacks or stroke should not take this drug. Ticagrelor is a reversible, oral ADP P2Y12 receptor antagonist that does not need metabolising; it has a short half-life of 12 hours and thus twice daily dosing is required. It is a potent drug but this benefit comes with an increased risk of bleeding and in a trial comparing Ticagrelor with Clopidogrel, higher rates of dyspnoea were observed in the ticagrelor group.

Abciximab, Eptifibatide and *Tirofiban* are potent antiplatelet agents, which bind to the GP IIb/IIIa receptor and are administered intravenously. Their use has been superseded by the thienopyrodines discussed above, but they remain useful in the acute stage for ACS patients who are clinically unstable or when there is slow flow or no reflow following PCI.

Anticoagulant drugs

Anticoagulation is used to prevent acute thrombus formation at the site of the plaque rupture or to prevent in-stent thrombosis after PCI. ACS patients should receive *Fondaparinux*, low molecular weight heparin (LMWH), *Bivalirudin* or unfractionated heparin (UFH). Newer indirect factor-Xa inhibitors (Fondaparinux) and direct thrombin inhibitors (Bivalirudin) inhibit thrombin mediated platelet activation and are now recommended in national guidance. *LMWH (Enoxaparin)* inhibits factor Xa and anti-thrombin and has a more sustained and predictable anticoagulant effect than UFH. It is administered subcutaneously twice daily and does not require aPTT monitoring. *UFH* exerts a number of effects; action on circulating antithrombin, which inactivates factor IIa, factor IXa and factor Xa. This leads to marked variation in patient response to therapy and monitoring is required with aPTT. High risk ACS patients may be commenced on a direct factor Xa inhibitor within 7 days of the acute event but Rivaroxaban is only currently licensed with Aspirin and Clopidogrel.

Reperfusion therapy

P-PCI provides a mechanical means of enlarging the lumen of the affected coronary artery by the insertion of a balloon-tipped catheter into the affected artery and inflation of the balloon to dilate the arterial lumen in a procedure known as balloon angioplasty. This is followed by deployment of a coronary artery stent and thrombectomy or atherectomy. The efficacy of P-PCI over fibrinolysis (thrombolysis) as the appropriate reperfusion treatment option in ACS is now indisputable. However, in rare circumstances when P-PCI is not immediately available (rural settings where transport times to PCI centres are prolonged), thrombolysis can be used if given within 30 minutes of acute presentation. Thrombolytics convert plasminogen to plasmin, which degrades fibrin and thrombus. Third-generation thrombolytics include *Reteplase* and *Tenecteplase*, both of which have enhanced fibrinolytic potency and can be given by bolus injection enhancing ease of administration. To prevent reocclusion of the infarct-related artery ancillary anticoagulant therapy such as Fondaparinux, LMWH or UFH should be given. Absolute contraindications to thrombolytic therapy include intracranial haemorrhage, uncontrolled hypertension or recent closed head or facial trauma. Practitioners should check the list of contraindications issued by the drug manufacturers.

Secondary prevention Beta-Blockers, ACE-inhibitors and Statins

Reduction in post-ACS mortality is achieved with the use of beta-blockers, ACE-I and statins.

Beta-blockers should be commenced as soon as possible after the ACS event. Beta-blockers such as *Bisoprolol* block the effect of catecholamines on adrenergic receptors in the myocardium, reducing myocardial contractility and slowing the heart rate. The beneficial effects are to decrease cardiac output, reduce myocardial oxygen demand and increase diastolic filling time hence augmenting coronary blood flow.

Angiotensin-converting enzyme inhibitors (ACE-I) block the conversion of angiotensin I to angiotensin II, a potent vasoconstrictor. ACE-I such as *Ramipril* have been shown to reduce mortality and left ventricle (LV) remodelling post ACS. Patients who cannot tolerate ACE-I can be given angiotensin receptor blockers (ARBs).

Statins such as *Atorvastatin* inhibit HMG CoA reductase production in the liver and lower LDL cholesterol. Unless contraindicated, all patients with ACS should take a statin to lower and then maintain a normal LDL cholesterol level.

Administration of an insulin infusion for patients presenting with hyperglycaemia during or immediately following an episode of ACS has been shown to reduce the risk of further cardiac events or death, even in patients not known to have diabetes.

Adherence and side-effects

Most patients with ACS will be taking at least 5 drugs: aspirin, thienopyridine, ACE-I, beta-blocker and statin. The importance of optimal secondary prevention to ensure long-term survival is evident, but the use of 5 drugs poses a challenge for patient adherence. Patients should be encouraged to persevere with all drugs, but also advised of any risks. Patients taking dual-antiplatelet therapy are advised to be vigilant for evidence of bleeding which will not resolve. Patients taking ACE-I should have renal function monitored regularly and patients taking statins should be advised of the possibility of long-term muscle pain. All patients should be referred for cardiac rehabilitation to optimise lifestyle gains. They should be advised and supported with smoking cessation, weight loss and increase in exercise levels if appropriate.

Acute heart failure

Acute heart failure is a life-threatening condition in which the patient experiences rapid onset of the symptoms associated with heart failure. Rapid assessment and treatment is necessary to ensure the comfort and safety of the patient. Several factors are known to trigger acute heart failure, such as acute coronary syndrome and tachyarrhythmia, which usually require additional treatments.

History

Acute heart failure may occur in response to the sudden onset of an acute cardiovascular event, such as acute coronary syndrome, aortic dissection, tachyarrhythmia or pulmonary embolus. However, many patients with chronic heart failure may experience an episode of acute decompensation, precipitated by new onset of infection, arrhythmia or non-adherence to prescribed medications or fluid and dietary salt restrictions.

Signs and symptoms

Paroxysmal nocturnal dyspnoea, orthopnoea, cough, peripheral oedema and weight gain are common symptoms associated with pulmonary congestion, caused by fluid overload. Dizziness, fatigue and confusion are symptoms associated with low cardiac output. Patients with acute heart failure often feel anxious and distressed.

Clinical signs include tachypnoea, hypoxaemia, use of respiratory accessory muscles and bilateral pulmonary crackles on auscultation. Sputum may appear white or pink and frothy. Hypoperfusion may cause hypotension, diaphoresis, cool extremities and oliguria and if associated with a systolic BP < 90 mmHg, cardiogenic shock is diagnosed. Additional signs include narrow pulse pressure, jugular venous distension, congested hepatomegaly and ascites.

In addition, the patient may experience symptoms and signs associated with the precipitating event, such as sepsis, tachyarrhythmia or acute coronary syndrome.

Assessment and investigations

Rapid assessment and history taking is necessary to establish a diagnosis of acute heart failure and to ascertain the cause of the episode. Patients should be closely monitored during the first hour, with regular observations and continuous pulse oximetry, cardiac monitoring and non-invasive haemodynamic monitoring. A record of urine output and fluid balance should be kept. Investigations should include a 12-lead ECG, chest X-ray and echocardiogram to ascertain the extent of cardiac dysfunction and identify the cause. Blood tests should include natriuretic peptides, such as B-type natriuretic peptides (BNP) and NT pro-BNP, cardiac troponin, urea, creatinine and electrolytes, as well as liver and thyroid function tests and arterial blood gas sampling. Once the patient is stable, their weight should be recorded.

Treatment

Patients with acute heart failure should be treated in a setting that provides close monitoring and rapid access to resuscitation equipment. The patient should be positioned upright in the high Fowler's position and high flow oxygen should be administered if the patient is hypoxaemic. Patients may be frightened and so reassurance is essential. Opiates may be required for patients in considerable distress but should be administered cautiously as bradycardia, hypotension or respiratory depression may result. Anxiolytics may be necessary to treat patients with delirium.

In patients diagnosed with acute heart failure with a systolic BP > 90 mmHg, intravenous diuretics, nitrates and continuous positive airway pressure (CPAP) can relieve pulmonary congestion and improve respiratory function. However, all three interventions should be administered with close monitoring as they could worsen hypotension and precipitate cardiogenic shock. Inotropic support is indicated in patients with severe hypoperfusion in the absence of hypovolaemia. Cautious administration is again necessary as inotropes can cause sinus tachycardia, myocardial ischaemia and arrhythmias. Ultrafiltration is an alternative intervention in patients with an acute exacerbation of chronic heart failure who no longer respond to diuretic therapy. Patients with acute heart failure may develop AF for which thromboembolic prophylaxis and digoxin are appropriate treatments.

Once haemodynamic stability is restored, patients diagnosed with chronic heart failure should be offered a range of treatments and lifestyle advice to minimise recurrence of symptoms, prevent acute exacerbations and optimise quality of life. ACE-Inhibitors (ACE-I) and beta-blockers have been demonstrated to reduce mortality and morbidity and the introduction of aldosterone inhibitors, such as Spironolactone or Eplerenone, also have proven benefits. Diuretics, such as Furosemide, Bumetanide or Metolazone, may be offered to control fluid retention. Recent data has revealed that a new drug, Sacubitril Valsartan, that combines a neprilysin inhibitor and angiotensin receptor blocker (ARB), may be a more effective alternative to an ACE-I in some patients with a reduced ejection fraction. Cardiac resynchronisation therapy, also known as bi-ventricular pacing, may additionally offer some improvement in symptoms for patients with a symptomatic heart failure.

Patients are encouraged to manage their condition themselves through careful monitoring and lifestyle adjustments. They should be advised to strictly limit salt and water intake to reduce weight and fluid gains. A cardiac rehabilitation programme provides education and support, as well as a supervised exercise programme, which has been shown to improve patients' exercise capacity, reduce hospital admissions and improve quality of life. Many patients frequently experience anxiety and depression for which self-help groups provide support for patients and their carers in learning to live with this long-term condition.

Aortic aneurysm

An aortic aneurysm is a localised dilatation of the thoracic or abdominal aorta resulting from weakening of all three layers of the arterial wall. An aneurysm is diagnosed when the diameter of the aorta is found to have increased by at least 50%. The most significant complications associated with aortic aneurysm are rupture or dissection, resulting in blood loss, hypotension and cardiac arrest.

History

Aortic aneurysms develop when the elastin fibres within the aorta degenerate as a result of ageing, hypertension or specific connective tissue disorders such as Marfan syndrome. Aortic aneurysms affecting the descending thoracic and abdominal aorta are strongly associated with atherosclerosis and cardiovascular risk factors, such as hypertension, dyslipidaemia, smoking and advancing age, which contribute to weakening of the vessel wall. A pseudoaneurysm (false aneurysm) occurs when blood passes from the lumen through a channel within the intima and medial layers and collects within the adventitia.

Signs and symptoms

Patients with aortic aneurysm are frequently asymptomatic. However, symptoms may occur if the aneurysm is large enough to compress adjacent structures, such as the trachea, bronchus or oesophagus resulting in stridor, hoarseness, dyspnoea, cough or dysphagia. Ascending aortic aneurysms may dilate the aortic valve, resulting in the symptoms associated with aortic regurgitation and heart failure. Rupture of an aortic aneurysm may occur with a slow leak or sudden burst, causing hypotension and tachycardia associated with profound blood loss and may result in cardiac arrest.

Assessment and investigations

Patients presenting with a ruptured aortic aneurysm will require rapid assessment and close monitoring prior to transfer for emergency surgery. Thoracic aortic aneurysm is often an incidental finding from investigations such as chest X-ray, echocardiogram, CT scan or MRI. Once identified, a CT scan will enable identification of the exact location and dimensions of the aneurysm, which will be used to guide the management of the patient. An aortogram may also be used to identify which arterial branches of the aorta are affected.

Treatment

Rapid surgical intervention is the only curative option for patients with ruptured aortic aneurysm. In the absence of rupture or dissection, treatment for patients is guided by the diameter of the aorta. The risk of rupture significantly increases as the aorta widens beyond 6 cm. Open surgical deployment with a prosthetic graft is recommended once the aortic diameter is more than 6 cm or if rupture has occurred. Thoracic Endovascular Aortic Repair (TEVAR) with a stent graft is an increasingly common alternative intervention. Close monitoring and conservative pharmacological blood pressure management to reduce the risk of rupture is recommended for patients with an aortic diameter of less than 6 cm and for those unsuitable for surgical intervention.

Aortic dissection

Aortic dissection occurs when a tear in the intimal layer of the aorta creates a false channel that permits blood flow into the tunica media. Aortic dissection is a life-threatening condition requiring emergency surgical intervention.

History

Thoracic aortic dissection occurs more frequently in men and is associated with advancing age, hypertension, Marfan syndrome and trauma. A classification system is used to specify the region of the aorta affected by the dissection. Stanford Type A dissection affects the ascending thoracic aorta, the most commonly affected region, which may extend to the aortic root, the aortic arch or the descending thoracic aorta. Stanford Type B dissections affect the descending thoracic aorta and may extend to the abdominal aorta.

Signs and symptoms

Aortic dissection is characterised by a 'tearing' or 'ripping' pain located either between the scapulae, associated with a type B dissection, or in the central chest region, suggesting type A dissection. The location of the pain may spread throughout the chest and back or to the abdomen if the dissection extends beyond the thoracic aorta. An array of additional symptoms, such as limb ischaemia and acute kidney injury, may emerge, dependent upon whether major arteries originating from the aorta are affected. For example, the patient may appear confused or with reduced level of consciousness if the left common carotid artery arising from the aortic arch is affected. Tachycardia and hypertension usually occur, initially due to the sympathetic response to pain or reduced renal perfusion, but will deteriorate if reduced myocardial perfusion or cardiac tamponade, associated with a type A dissection, occur.

Assessment and investigations

Rapid, systematic assessment of the patient with suspected aortic dissection is required to aid diagnosis and selection of an appropriate treatment strategy. Cardiovascular assessment should include cardiac monitoring, regular pulse assessment and blood pressure recordings from both arms, which may be different if the dissection originates in the aortic arch. Acute coronary syndrome should be rapidly ruled out using comprehensive chest pain assessment and serial 12-lead ECGs. It should be noted that ST-segment elevation, usually affecting the inferior leads, may be evident if right coronary arterial perfusion is affected in type A aortic dissection. A urinary catheter should be inserted to facilitate accurate fluid balance monitoring. Serum bloods should include full blood count, urea and electrolytes, troponin, clotting screen and cross-match prior to surgery. A chest X-ray may reveal a widened mediastinum associated with type A dissection; CT, MRI or transoesophageal echocardiogram will confirm the presence of aortic dissection.

Treatment

Preventing progression of the dissection should be prioritised in the management of both type A and type B aortic dissection, by maintaining the patient's systolic blood pressure between 100–120 mmHg with beta-blockers and intravenous vasodilator infusions such as glyceryl trinitrate (GTN). Emergency cardiac surgery is usually necessary for patients with type A dissection to either repair or replace the damaged intimal layer with a prosthetic graft, although research is on-going into the role of Thoracic Endovascular Aortic Repair (TEVAR) to treat dissection. Conservative medical therapy alone may be recommended for patients with type B dissection, unless complications affecting major arterial branches necessitate urgent endovascular stenting or surgical repair.

Aortic regurgitation

Aortic regurgitation (AR) is reflux of blood from the aorta into the left ventricle (LV) across the leaking aortic valve during diastole. This results in pressure and volume overload in the LV, which hypertrophies to accommodate the regurgitation, the stroke volume increases and the major arteries become visibly pulsatile. As the disease progresses LV end diastolic pressure (LVEDP) rises and the increased LV mass becomes increasingly inefficient with reduced coronary perfusion. Increased LVEDP may also cause mitral regurgitation and subsequent left atrial dilatation, increased pulmonary pressure and symptoms of atrial arrhythmias and left ventricular failure (LVF).

History

AR may be caused by chronic untreated hypertension, abnormalities of the aortic valve cusps (bicuspid aortic valve, endocarditis or rheumatic heart disease) or diseases of the aortic root (Marfan syndrome, syphilis, aneurysm or dissection). Chronic AR may develop over many years and during this period the patient may be asymptomatic. It is only when the compensatory mechanisms fail that LV dysfunction leads to a reduction in left ventricular ejection fraction. In acute AR, due to aortic dissection or infective endocarditis, the LV is of normal size and cannot cope with the increased volume. LVF develops rapidly and raised left atrial and pulmonary capillary pressure leads to catastrophic pulmonary oedema.

Signs and symptoms

In chronic AR, the patient may have an awareness of the heart beat or palpitations on exertion, during stress or when lying on the left side. This may also be associated with a pounding sensation in the head. As the disease progresses and LVF ensues, symptoms of dyspnoea, paroxysmal nocturnal dyspnoea, fatigue and weakness will develop. Clinical signs in AR are due to the hyper-dynamic circulation; a large volume or 'collapsing pulse', bounding peripheral pulses, a widened pulse pressure and a displaced heaving apex beat. There may be an early diastolic murmur, a systolic murmur and bilateral inspiratory crackles with pulmonary oedema. Patients may develop angina due to increased LV mass and reduced coronary perfusion. The 12-lead ECG may show LV hypertrophy, left axis deviation and left ventricular strain pattern.

Acute AR presents with a sudden onset of heart failure and reduced cardiac output. Tachycardia, hypotension, cardiovascular collapse and cardiogenic shock all require urgent intervention.

Assessment and investigations

Acute AR requires urgent assessment and treatment of the patient. Airway and respiratory assessment including rate, depth, breathing pattern and peripheral oxygen monitoring should be undertaken.

Heart and breath sounds, pulse, blood pressure and cardiac rhythm should be monitored for cardiogenic shock, atrial and ventricular arrhythmias and evidence of heart failure. A 12-lead ECG may demonstrate LV hypertrophy and myocardial ischaemia; ACS should be excluded. An echocardiogram will confirm AR as the cause of the patient's symptoms and a chest X-ray will evaluate pulmonary oedema and cardiomegaly. Arterial blood gases will be required, venous samples will assess urea and electrolytes (U&Es), full blood count (FBC), troponin, B-type natriuretic peptides (BNP) and glucose levels. Fluid balance and weight should be monitored and fluid restrictions may be required.

Treatment
In the acute phase, patients may need oxygen therapy and treatment with vasodilators and inotropes. In chronic AR, systolic blood pressure is controlled with ACE inhibitors or calcium channel blockers. Timing of aortic valve/root replacement or repair is crucial and may be performed before the patient becomes symptomatic to avoid development of LV dysfunction.

Aortic stenosis

Aortic stenosis (AS) occurs when the leaflets (cusps) of the aortic valve become stiffened. During ventricular systole, the opening of the valve is significantly impeded, reducing stroke volume and eventually resulting in heart failure.

History

The most common cause of AS is age-related sclerosis, which causes the cusps to stiffen and fuse together, preventing the valve from opening fully during left ventricular systole. Early detection of AS is difficult as the patient will not usually experience symptoms until the disease is in the advanced stages, when the valve orifice has been reduced to approximately one-third of its normal size. Less commonly, AS can occur with a congenital bicuspid aortic valve or as a result of streptococcal infection in childhood (rheumatic fever). AS is also known to be a rare form of congenital heart disease.

Signs and symptoms

AS produces a triad of classic clinical symptoms, usually occurring on exertion: dyspnoea, chest pain, pre-syncope or syncope. The patient may experience fatigue as well as other symptoms caused by heart failure, such as ankle swelling and palpitations, which may be due to atrial or ventricular arrhythmias. AS can cause sudden cardiac death.

Clinical signs include a slow rising, low volume pulse and signs associated with heart failure, including jugular venous distension (JVD) and peripheral oedema. On auscultation, AS will produce an ejection systolic murmur and possibly an ejection systolic click; a soft 2nd heart sound, S3 and bilateral (inspiratory/expiratory) crackles associated with pulmonary oedema. The 12-lead ECG may show evidence of left ventricular hypertrophy, atrial enlargement, left anterior fascicular block or left bundle branch block.

Assessment and investigations

Initial assessment of the patient should prioritise baseline observations, continuous cardiac monitoring, chest pain assessment and 12-lead ECG to rapidly rule out acute coronary syndrome as the cause of the symptoms. The patient should be assessed for the signs of heart failure and a chest X-ray and blood samples taken to assess for renal dysfunction, including estimated glomerular filtration rate (eGFR), electrolyte imbalance, full blood count, troponin and B-type natriuretic peptides (BNP). A fluid balance chart should be commenced immediately and the patient may require a urinary catheter. Once stable, the patient should be weighed daily. An echocardiogram will establish the diagnosis of AS and measure the LV ejection fraction.

An angiogram will assess the severity of the AS by measuring the difference in systolic pressure between the left ventricle (LV) and aorta (gradient).

Treatment

The treatment for hypoxia, dyspnoea, chest pain or anxiety should be prioritised initially with bed rest, oxygen therapy, frusemide and morphine, with an anti-emetic if required. Nitrates should be avoided due to the vasodilator effect that can reduce ventricular preload, which would further decrease cardiac output. Electrolyte imbalance should be corrected to prevent possible arrhythmias. The patient should be encouraged to rest to minimise exertion and prevent symptoms. Most patients with symptomatic AS will require surgical intervention urgently. Aortic valve replacement surgery remains the mainstay of treatment but if the patient is unsuitable for surgery, transcutaneous aortic valve implantation (TAVI) is an effective alternative. Conservative management includes avoidance of strenuous exercise and pharmacological therapy including beta-blockers or calcium channel blockers to reduce myocardial work.

Arrhythmogenic right ventricular cardiomyopathy

Arrhythmogenic right ventricular cardiomyopathy (ARVC) or dysplasia (ARVD) is a rare, inherited form of cardiomyopathy in which heart failure is caused by fibro-fatty replacement of myocytes, predominantly within the right ventricle (RV). The risk of ventricular arrhythmias is increased, principally on exertion and therefore ARVC is a known cause of sudden cardiac death.

History

ARVC is an autosomal dominant inherited condition in which genetic mutation causes damage to the proteins within the desmosome, the bridge that joins myocytes together. As the desmosome weakens, the myocytes separate, allowing deposition of adipose and fibrous tissue, forming scar tissue. This process is thought to accelerate with strenuous exertion. Structural changes to the RV will initially be minimal, usually affecting the inflow, outflow and apical regions. Later, the fibro-fatty tissue may extend to all regions of the RV, causing dilatation and systolic dysfunction. Some patients may eventually develop left ventricular involvement.

Signs and symptoms

The clinical features of ARVC develop over time, although disease progression is variable among patients and some patients remain asymptomatic. Premature ventricular contractions (PVCs), and non-sustained and sustained VT may occur at any stage of the condition; the first presentation may be cardiac arrest, usually following strenuous activity. ARVC should be considered in patients presenting with right ventricular outflow tract (RVOT) tachycardia (left bundle branch block pattern with a rightward mean QRS axis). Patients may also describe symptoms associated with heart failure or syncope.

Assessments and investigations

Approximately 30–50% of patients with ARVC have a family history of the condition. Currently there is no single test to identify AVRC; genetic testing will only be helpful in some cases. International criteria are used to diagnose AVRC using familial, histological, electrocardiographical and structural data. The 12-lead ECG may reveal QRS prolongation or Epsilon waves. Late potentials may be evident on the signal-averaged ECG. 24-hour Holter monitoring and exercise testing should be used to identify the occurrence of ventricular arrhythmias. An echocardiogram may reveal RV dilatation and reduced RV ejection fraction with normal LV function. Invasive diagnostic tests include electrophysiology studies, right ventriculogram and endomyocardial biopsy.

Treatment

The treatment for ARVC aims to prevent the occurrence of life-threatening arrhythmias and to limit the extent of right ventricular systolic dysfunction. Pharmacological therapy includes anti-arrhythmic agents such as beta blockers or amiodarone to prevent arrhythmias. The patient may be offered radio-frequency ablation and an implantable cardioverter defibrillator (ICD) to prevent or treat ventricular arrhythmias. ACE-inhibitors may be prescribed to minimise systolic dysfunction. Close relatives of the patient should be offered genetic counselling prior to screening for ARVC.

Atrial fibrillation

Atrial fibrillation (AF) is a commonly occurring arrhythmia that may result in acute heart failure or stroke. AF occurs when multiple, rapid re-entry circuits cause the atria to fibrillate at a rate of 300–600 bpm. The AV node protects the ventricles by restricting the conduction of impulses through to the ventricles. This results in an irregular, narrow QRS complex arrhythmia with a ventricular rate between 30 and 180 bpm. AF may be paroxysmal or permanent.

History

AF is the most common sustained arrhythmia affecting individuals over 65 years of age and is frequently idiopathic in origin. Reversible causes of AF include hypoxia, chest infections, excess alcohol or caffeine consumption, electrolyte imbalance, emotional stress, fluid overload or drugs that can induce tachycardia, for example Salbutamol. AF can also be caused by acute exacerbation of heart failure and is strongly associated with conditions that dilate the atria, such as mitral valve regurgitation, dilated cardiomyopathy or hypertension. AF commonly occurs after cardiac surgery.

Signs and symptoms

The patient may present with sudden onset of palpitations, dyspnoea, chest pain, fatigue, pre-syncopal or syncopal symptoms, or other signs associated with heart failure. The patient's pulse will be irregular, weak and thready on palpation. The diagnosis will be made from the cardiac monitor, 12-lead ECG or 24-hour tape that will typically show an irregular rhythm at a rate of 30–180 bpm with a normal duration QRS complex (<100 ms) (unless bundle branch block is present). No discernible P waves will be evident, although fibrillatory waves may be visible (Figure 12.1).

AF is associated with a high risk of stroke due to stasis and coagulation of blood within the fibrillating atria. If sustained for more than 48 hours, thrombus formation will occur, particularly within the left atrial appendage from which emboli could be displaced into the systemic circulation. This risk is increased when sinus rhythm is restored.

Assessment and investigations

Initial systematic assessment of a patient with new onset AF should use the ABCDE approach and include a 12-lead ECG. Continuous

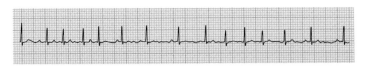

Figure 12.1 Atrial fibrillation (AF) as seen in lead II.

cardiac monitoring, regular observations and fluid balance measurements are necessary to monitor for acute deterioration. Establishing the cause of AF should be prioritised. Serum blood tests should be taken to identify electrolyte imbalance and renal dysfunction and record a clotting screen. Individual risk assessment should be conducted using the 'CHA$_2$DS$_2$-VASc' score to establish risk of thromboembolism, offset against the risk of bleeding associated with anti-coagulant therapy using the 'HAS-BLED' score.

Treatment

Emergency treatment will be required for the patient who becomes haemodynamically unstable with AF. This will usually be rapid direct current cardioversion (DCCV) unless the ventricular response is very slow, in which case the patient will require transcutaneous pacing. Beta-blockers or calcium channel blockers are suitable drug treatments to slow the ventricular response rate in fast AF; Digoxin is preferred in patients with heart failure. Amiodarone is recommended where cardioversion is sought, for example post-cardiac surgery. Elective DCCV, radio-frequency and cryoablation are therapeutic options if AF persists.

Anti-coagulation should be considered for all patients with paroxysmal or permanent AF, to reduce the risk of thromboembolic complications such as stroke. During the acute phase, anti-thrombin therapy, such as low molecular weight heparin, should be initiated and continued until therapeutic levels of anti-coagulation are established. Warfarin may be prescribed for this or, alternatively, a non-vitamin K oral anticoagulant (NOAC), such as Rivaroxaban, may be suitable, although not recommended for patients with AF caused by valve disease. Aspirin does not protect against the thromboembolic risk and is therefore not recommended.

Atrial flutter

Atrial flutter is a relatively uncommon arrhythmia that may result in acute heart failure or stroke. Atrial flutter occurs when an ectopic atrial site, usually close to the atrio-ventricular (AV) node, generates regular impulses at a rate of 300/min. The rhythm is the result of either increased automaticity or a rapid macro re-entry circuit in the atria. The atrial flutter completely suppresses the activity of the sino-atrial (SA) node. The ectopic atrial pacemaker fires rapidly and the series of atrial impulses create a waveform with a characteristic saw-tooth appearance called an F wave. The AV node will have a decremental effect on the rapid F wave rate, blocking conduction to the ventricles in a ratio of 2:1, 3:1 or 4:1. This results in a narrow, complex, regular rhythm of 150, 100 or 75 bpm respectively. There may also be variable conduction through the AV node, resulting in an irregular QRS rate. Atrial flutter may be paroxysmal or permanent.

History

Atrial flutter, whilst relatively rare, has many reversible causes including hypoxia, chest infections, excess alcohol or caffeine consumption, electrolyte imbalance, emotional stress, fluid overload or use of drugs that can induce tachycardia, for example Salbutamol. Atrial flutter can occur during acute heart failure and is strongly associated with conditions that dilate the atria, such as mitral valve regurgitation, dilated cardiomyopathy or hypertension. Atrial flutter commonly occurs after cardiac surgery.

Signs and symptoms

A patient with an acute onset of atrial flutter may present in a collapsed state with signs of shock, particularly if the conduction rate is 2:1 or if the patient has pre-existing ventricular dysfunction. A sudden onset of atrial flutter may cause palpitations, anxiety, dyspnoea, chest pain and syncope or signs of heart failure. Atrial dysfunction results in blood stasis and the potential for atrial thrombus, which may embolise resulting in pulmonary embolus or stroke. The diagnosis will be made from the ECG, which will typically show a regular, narrow complex QRS with the characteristic saw-tooth flutter waves known as F waves (Figure 13.1). In Lead II, a typical F wave has an inverted negative deflection reflecting abnormal atrial depolarisation followed by a positive F wave deflection reflecting atrial repolarisation.

Assessment and investigations

Initial systematic assessment of a patient with new onset atrial flutter should use the ABCDE approach and include a 12-lead ECG and SpO_2 monitoring. Continuous cardiac monitoring, regular vital signs and

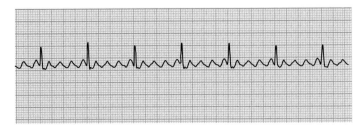

Figure 13.1 Atrial flutter.

fluid balance measurements are necessary to monitor for acute deterioration. Serum blood tests should be taken to identify electrolyte imbalance, renal dysfunction and to record a clotting screen. The risks of thromboembolism offset against the risk of bleeding associated with anti-coagulant therapy should be assessed using 'CHA$_2$DS$_2$-VASc' and 'HAS-BLED' risk scores. Sudden resumption of sinus rhythm increases the risk of stroke.

Treatment
The treatment depends on the haemodynamic consequences of the arrhythmia. A ventricular rate of 150 bpm will often cause rapid collapse and deterioration in most patients. Emergency treatment is directed to restoring sinus rhythm using direct current (DC) cardioversion. If the patient has a ventricular rate of less than 150 bpm and is not haemodynamically compromised, acute pharmacological cardioversion using class 1c (flecainide) or class III (Sotalol or Amiodarone) antiarrhythmic drugs can be used. Patients who have been in atrial flutter longer than 48 hours should be anticoagulated and cardioversion delayed until the thromboembolic risk has reduced. Recurrent atrial flutter can be prevented by Sotalol or Amiodarone to control the ventricular rate, although the treatment of choice for recurrence is catheter ablation to permanently interrupt the atrial re-entry circuit.

Brugada syndrome

Brugada syndrome is an autosomal dominant ion-channelopathy, which occurs in structurally normal hearts. The condition may only manifest when the patient presents with an aborted sudden cardiac death, but pre-morbid symptoms may include syncope, palpitations and seizures. The most common cardiac arrhythmia is polymorphic ventricular tachycardia (VT), which may deteriorate to ventricular fibrillation. It is a leading cause of sudden cardiac death in healthy individuals.

History

The syndrome was first described in 1992, by the Brugada brothers, as a distinct clinical and electrocardiographic syndrome following investigation of eight patients who had survived an out-of-hospital cardiac arrest and who were found to have characteristic ECG abnormalities. This was subsequently linked to a high incidence of sudden cardiac deaths in the Philippines and Thailand, where syndromes had been respectively described as 'bangungut' (to rise and scream in the night) and 'lai tai' (death during sleeping). In 1998, the mutation of the sodium channel gene 5A (SCN5A) was identified and the hereditary nature of the syndrome was confirmed.

Signs and symptoms

There is a wide phenotype variation and some patients may be asymptomatic and only diagnosed on routine 12-lead ECG examination. Some patients may suffer with palpitations and syncope; the underlying arrhythmia is polymorphic VT. Many patients die during sleep and death may be preceded by chest pain, seizures, loss of bladder control and laboured breathing. The first arrhythmic events tend to occur around 40 years of age, but may occur between 1 and 70 years.

Assessment and investigations

The diagnosis is aided by patient and family history, electrocardiogram and genetic testing. Patients are normally fit and healthy and hence physical examination will be normal. The 12-lead ECG presentation is characterised by down-sloping ST-segment elevation in V_1–V_3 with a right bundle branch block pattern (Figure 14.1). In patients with a 'concealed form' of Brugada Syndrome, the ECG pattern or arrhythmia may only be revealed after provocation during an electrophysiological study, a VT stimulation study or the administration of Ajmaline. Genetic testing may identify the SCN5A gene and help in predictive testing for other family members.

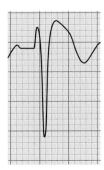

Figure 14.1 Brugada Sign: down-sloping ST elevation with right bundle branch block pattern (V_1).

Treatment
Anti-arrhythmic drug therapy is not useful in Brugada syndrome and the only effective treatment is implantation of an internal implantable cardioverter defibrillator (ICD). Genetic testing and counselling is essential for any family members affected.

Cardiac arrest

Cardiac arrest is defined as sudden cessation of effective systemic blood flow due to failure of cardiac contraction. It is rapidly accompanied by absent respiratory effort and loss of consciousness. If not treated, death will occur within minutes.

History

Most sudden unexpected deaths are due to cardiac arrest, which is preceded by cardiac symptom onset. The underlying arrhythmias are ventricular fibrillation or ventricular tachycardia; rarely the presentation may be extreme bradycardia or asystole. Cardiac arrest is usually caused by underlying cardiac conditions such as acute coronary syndrome, aneurysm, cardiomyopathy, electrophysiological abnormalities, infective heart disease or valvular heart disease. Other causes include pulmonary embolism, cerebral or subarachnoid haemorrhage, electrolyte or metabolic disturbances.

Assessment

Ensure it is safe to approach the patient and assess responsiveness by shaking him and shouting in his ear. Open the patient's airway by placing the patient on his back, flexing the neck and extending the head using the 'head tilt – chin lift' method. Rapidly check (no more than 10 seconds) if the patient is breathing by looking for chest movement, listening at the mouth for breath sounds and feeling for air on your cheek. At the same time, check for presence of the carotid pulse. If the patient is unresponsive and there are no other signs of life, help should be sought and basic life support commenced. Apply personal protective clothing as soon as possible and especially if the patient has a known infective condition.

Treatment

The Resuscitation Council (UK) guidance was issued in 2015 and is approved by the National Institute of Health and Care Excellence. The 'Chain of Survival' (Figure 15.1) includes early recognition of warning signs, early activation of emergency services, early basic life support including cardiopulmonary resuscitation (CPR), early defibrillation and early Advanced Cardiac Life Support (ACLS). When a patient is found to be in cardiac arrest, the in-hospital resuscitation team or emergency services should be summoned immediately.

CPR should be commenced, in cycles of 30 regular chest compressions, at a rate of 100–120/min, depressing the sternum by 5–6 cm, followed by 2 effective breaths. As soon as possible, the

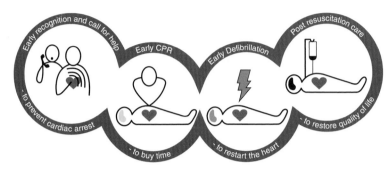

Figure 15.1 The Chain of Survival.

patient should be attached to a defibrillator/monitor to assess cardiac rhythm. If the patient has a 'shockable rhythm' (ventricular tachycardia or ventricular fibrillation) an unsynchronised shock of 150–200 J biphasic (360 J monophasic) should be delivered followed immediately by 2 minutes of CPR. If the patient remains in ventricular tachycardia/ventricular fibrillation (VT/VF), this cycle of CPR and shocks should be repeated. Amiodarone should be administered after the third shock. If the patient has a 'non-shockable rhythm', i.e. asystole or pulseless electrical activity (PEA), continuous CPR should be administered and the rhythm reassessed every 2 minutes.

Vascular access should be established promptly to facilitate administration of adrenaline every 3–5 minutes. Oxygen delivery should be maintained, although the patient's airway may need to be secured using endotracheal intubation or a supraglottic airway.

Treatable causes should be considered using the 4 'H's' (Hypoxia, Hypovolaemia, Hyper/Hypokalaemia and Hypothermia) and 4 'T's' (Thromboembolism, Tension Pneumothorax, Tamponade and Toxins). Percutaneous coronary intervention should be expedited for cardiac causes, even if the patient remains in cardiac arrest.

On return of spontaneous circulation, the patient should be systematically assessed and closely monitored using the ABCDE approach and a 12-lead ECG recorded. Patients may require ventilator support, necessitating transfer to an intensive care setting. Targeted temperature management may be implemented, although this remains disputable.

Cardiac arrhythmias: treatment and interventions

Cardiac arrhythmias can be treated using a variety of medications and devices that can control the rate of the rhythm, address the underlying cause of the arrhythmia or return the heart to a stable rhythm.

Mechanisms of arrhythmias

Anti-arrhythmic drugs are used to treat cardiac arrhythmias that are caused by three mechanisms affecting the action potential of cardiac myocytes: enhanced automaticity, triggered activity and re-entry.

Enhanced automaticity refers to the accelerated activation of depolarisation that can occur in both pacemaker cells and cardiac myocytes at the end of phase 4 of the action potential. Sinus tachycardia can occur when adrenaline enhances the normal automaticity of the sino-atrial (SA) node. Cardiac disease, drugs and low potassium levels may accelerate depolarisation of cardiac myocytes, referred to as enhanced abnormal automaticity.

Triggered activity can occur when the action potential of cardiac myocytes fails to return to the resting membrane potential of $-90\,mV$ during phase 3. Early or delayed after-depolarisations can occur when the transmembrane potential oscillates around the threshold potential of approximately $-70\,mV$. Myocardial damage can cause early after-depolarisations that initiate ventricular arrhythmias, including Torsades de Pointes.

Re-entry mechanisms can cause tachyarrhythmias when an ectopic beat causes activation of two pathways within a ring of tissue: one that is refractory, as it has recently depolarised and is slow to repolarise (α), and another pathway that is slow to depolarise (β) but is ready to be activated due to fast repolarisation. If the ectopic beat is conducted slowly down the β pathway, the α pathway may be ready to be activated, conducting the impulse back up to the tissue above. This re-entry circuit results in a circus movement tachycardia, such as supraventricular tachycardia (SVT) or ventricular tachycardia (VT).

Anti-arrhythmic drugs

Anti-arrhythmic drugs modify cardiac conduction and are categorised within the Vaughan Williams classification based on their primary effect on the cardiac action potential. As well as treating arrhythmias, these drugs can be pro-arrhythmic and reduce ventricular contractility and therefore must be administered with caution.

Class I

Class I anti-arrhythmic drugs reduce the rate of sodium entry into the cell during depolarisation (phase 0) to prevent tachyarrhythmias. Drugs in this class should not be offered to patients with structural heart disease, as they are associated with increased mortality. Administration of these drugs is usually initiated under close cardiac monitoring in a hospital setting:

Class I drugs are further stratified into 3 subtypes:

- Class Ia drugs, such as disopyramide, additionally prolong the refractory period of the action potential, increasing the QT interval.
- Class Ib drugs, such as Lidocaine, shorten the refractory period and have no effect on the QT interval.
- Class Ic agents, such as Flecainide, have minimal effect on the refractory period but severely depress sodium entry into the cell.

Class II

Beta-blockers, or β-adrenergic receptor antagonists, are categorised as Class II anti-arrhythmic drugs. Beta-blockers limit the effect of catecholamines in phase 4 of the cardiac action potential, particularly affecting nodal tissue. Cardioselective beta-blockers include Metoprolol and Bisoprolol. Beta-blockers are effective for ventricular rate control in patients with fast atrial fibrillation due to their depressant effect on atrio-ventricular (AV) nodal conduction. However, they may also cause hypotension, as well as numerous other side-effects such as fatigue, and are not recommended for use in patients with asthma or chronic obstructive pulmonary disease (COPD).

Class III

Class III anti-arrhythmic drugs slow the re-entry of potassium into the cell during phase 3 of the action potential, resulting in prolongation of the refractory period and hence the QT interval. Sotalol and Amiodarone are considered to be 'mixed class', as Sotalol is also a beta-blocker, and amiodarone additionally affects the sodium and calcium channels. Amiodarone is indicated for both atrial and ventricular arrhythmias, even in patients with structural heart disease. However, it is associated with numerous serious side-effects that include pulmonary fibrosis.

Class IV

Class IV anti-arrhythmic drugs are the non-dihydropyridine calcium channel blockers (CCBs), such as Verapamil. These drugs prolong the refractory period of the AV node and reduce myocardial contractility, by slowing the influx of calcium into the cell during phase 2 of the action potential. CCBs may be suitable for patients with atrial arrhythmias and SVTs, although due to their negative inotropic effect, they may cause hypotension and should consequently be administered with caution.

Other drug treatments for arrhythmias

Certain drugs used to treat arrhythmias, such as Digoxin, Adenosine and Isoprenaline are not included this classification, as they do not affect the cardiac action potential.

Digoxin will reduce the ventricular rate in atrial arrhythmias and is often indicated in patients with atrial fibrillation and heart failure. Adenosine causes rapid, transient blockade of the AV node that is useful for treating patients with SVTs caused by re-entry mechanisms. Isoprenaline is a beta-adrenergic receptor agonist administered to increase the rate of depolarisation of the SA node.

Anti-coagulation, using Warfarin or a non-vitamin K oral anti-coagulant (NOAC), such as Rivaroxaban, may be indicated for stroke prevention in patients with atrial arrhythmias.

Therapeutic procedures for cardiac arrhythmias

A range of therapeutic procedures is available to treat patients who experience symptoms associated with cardiac arrhythmias.

Pacing

Cardiac pacing is primarily used to augment cardiac output by increasing heart rate in patients experiencing symptomatic bradyarrhythmia. When the patient is haemodynamically compromised, emergency cardiac pacing can be delivered using transcutaneous pacing controlled by an Automated External Defibrillator (AED) or via a transvenous pacing wire advanced into the right ventricle and connected to an external pulse generator. Epicardial pacing may be suitable for patients immediately following cardiac surgery.

When a permanent pacemaker is required, a small device is inserted into a subpectoral pocket, with one or two electrodes advanced into the right atrium and/or right ventricle to deliver single or dual chamber pacing. The pacemaker is capable of sensing underlying cardiac activity and delivering a small electrical current to trigger depolarisation when required to maintain a safe heart rate. Many permanent pacemakers are rate-responsive to facilitate adjustment of the patient's heart rate based on their level of exertion. Recent advances in technology have led to the development of wireless pacemakers.

Synchronised direct current cardioversion

Patients who become severely haemodynamically unstable due to the sudden onset of tachyarrhythmias may require synchronised direct current cardioversion (DCCV) to restore sinus rhythm. This involves a transthoracic electric shock that is timed by the defibrillator to coincide with the QRS complex, to avoid delivering the shock during ventricular repolarisation (T wave), which can induce the 'R on T' phenomenon that can trigger Torsades de Pointes or ventricular fibrillation. Cardioversion should be conducted while the patient is under sedation with appropriate airway management.

Catheter ablation

Radio-frequency ablation and cryoablation are invasive percutaneous interventions used for symptomatic tachyarrhythmias. The origin of the arrhythmia must first be established before a catheter is advanced via the femoral circulation to the site where radiofrequency waves or cryotherapy is delivered to destroy the tissue that triggers the arrhythmia. This treatment is particularly useful for arrhythmias caused by a re-entry mechanism such as A-V re-entry tachycardia (AVRT), A-V nodal re-entry tachycardia (AVNRT) and atrial flutter. Ablation may also be administered during cardiac surgery, particularly for atrial fibrillation.

Implantable Cardioverter Defibrillators (ICDs)

Implantable Cardioverter Defibrillators (ICDs) may be offered to patients who have life-threatening ventricular arrhythmias. A small device is implanted in a sub-pectoral pocket, from which electrodes are advanced into the right atrium and right ventricle. The ICD has the same capabilities as a permanent pacemaker, but in addition can detect and respond to tachyarrhythmias. The response is individually programmed within each ICD, usually involving initial anti-tachycardia pacing followed by a series of electrical shocks until sinus rhythm is restored. This may be extremely uncomfortable for the patient, who may lose consciousness during the event.

Cardiac resynchronisation therapy (CRT)

Cardiac resynchronisation therapy (CRT) may be offered to patients with advanced heart failure to optimise left ventricular function. CRT-P refers to the use of biventricular pacing that requires placement of three electrodes. The right atrial and ventricular electrodes facilitate dual chamber, rate-responsive pacing. An additional electrode activates the left ventricle from its position in the coronary sinus, accessed via the right atrium. Stimulation and depolarisation of the three chambers is individually timed to optimise ventricular diastolic and systolic function. A defibrillator function may be added to the device for patients at risk of VT associated with heart failure (CRT-D).

Cardiogenic shock

Cardiogenic shock is a severe form of acute heart failure, diagnosed when the patient shows signs of organ hypoperfusion, such as cyanosis, confusion and oliguria, in the absence of hypovolaemia, with a systolic blood pressure below 90 mmHg.

History

Cardiogenic shock usually occurs immediately following an acute cardiovascular event, such as acute coronary syndrome (ACS), tachyarrhythmia, myocarditis, thoracic aortic dissection or pulmonary embolus.

Signs and symptoms

Patients in cardiogenic shock present with symptoms associated with acute heart failure, including severe dyspnoea, ankle swelling and reduced level of consciousness. Peripheral and central pulse assessment will usually reveal tachycardia and jugular venous distension. Systolic blood pressure will be less than 90 mmHg; pulse pressure and mean arterial pressure are likely to be low, indicating reduced stroke volume and poor organ perfusion. Cardiorespiratory auscultation may reveal pulmonary crackles and third and fourth heart sounds. Signs of peripheral and central cyanosis may be present, such as cool, clammy skin that is mottled in appearance. Peripheral oedema is highly likely to be present.

Assessment and investigations

Patients with suspected cardiogenic shock should undergo rapid assessment and should be cared for in a high dependency environment. Observations should include assessment of airway, respiratory rate, depth and use of accessory muscles alongside continuous pulse oximetry. The patient should be commenced on continuous 3-, 5- or 12-lead cardiac monitoring. Insertion of an arterial line will provide continuous mean arterial pressure monitoring and permit regular arterial blood gas analysis. Central venous cannulation is useful for both invasive haemodynamic monitoring and inotropic drug administration. An echocardiogram should be conducted to establish the extent of ventricular dysfunction. A urinary catheter should be inserted and fluid balance closely monitored. A blood glucose level should be recorded and serum blood samples taken for natriuretic peptides, troponins, urea and electrolytes, lactate, C-reactive protein (CRP), D-dimer, liver function and thyroid function tests, full blood count and a clotting screen. A 12-lead ECG should be recorded promptly to rule out ACS as the cause of cardiogenic shock. If ACS is suspected, patients should have immediate coronary angiography, followed by primary percutaneous coronary intervention (PCI), if indicated.

Treatment

The aim of treatment for patients in cardiogenic shock is to improve organ perfusion by improving cardiac output and blood pressure. Administration of intravenous inotropes such as Dobutamine, and vasopressors such as Norepinephrine, may improve mean arterial pressure but will also induce tachycardia, which may prove detrimental. These drugs may be combined if there is insufficient response or insertion of an intra-aortic balloon pump may provide an alternative means of improving organ perfusion. Mechanical devices, such as the left ventricular assist device, can provide a bridge to cardiac transplantation or provide symptomatic relief for patients with end-stage heart failure.

Dilated cardiomyopathy

Dilated cardiomyopathy (DCM) refers to a spectrum of myocardial disorders resulting in ventricular dilatation and systolic impairment. DCM is the most common type of cardiomyopathy and causes significant morbidity and mortality; DCM is a major cause of sudden cardiac death and is also the most frequent cause of heart failure.

History

There are multiple aetiologies for DCM including idiopathic, familial (genetic), viral, toxic, alcoholic or ischaemic. Familial (genetic) DCM is caused by mutations in the structural proteins which comprise the cardiac myocytes. Ischaemic DCM is the result of the remodelling process of the left ventricle in response to injury, with a consequent reduction in ejection fraction. Toxins, such as anti-cancer therapies (anthracyclines), alcohol and infections (viral, bacterial, fungal or parasitic) are also implicated in damage to the contractile processes in the heart. Autoimmune and infiltrative causes, such as systemic lupus erythematosus or amyloidosis, are rare. Pathologically, there is an increase in myocardial mass and a reduction in ventricular wall thickness. The heart becomes globular in shape with diffuse ventricular dilatation, atrial enlargement, thrombus formation in the atrial appendages and development of an intraventricular conduction delay.

Signs and symptoms

Patients with DCM may present with symptoms of heart failure, arrhythmias, conduction defects (bundle branch blocks), thromboembolism or sudden death. Common features are fatigue, breathlessness, chest pain, palpitations and fluid overload. Syncope or palpitations at rest are worrying symptoms as they may predict sudden cardiac death. Onset of symptoms may be slow and insidious or sudden and acute, dependent on the aetiology. Mitral regurgitation is a common feature in DCM and patients may present with a left ventricular heave and a pan-systolic murmur on auscultation.

Assessment and investigations

Careful history taking is essential to establish the aetiology and to identify reversible and secondary causes. Risk factors, such as excessive use of alcohol, past medical history of cancer or recent febrile events, may point to the aetiology. Patients with high risk symptoms, such as syncope or palpitations on exertion, should be treated with a high index of suspicion.

Vital signs should be carried out to evaluate the temperature (infectious causes), heart rate and rhythm (atrial and ventricular arrhythmias), respiratory rate and oxygen saturation (heart failure). Physical examination will include palpation of the heart for apical thrill, left ventricular heave and auscultation of the heart for evidence of mitral regurgitation. A 12-lead ECG should be performed and may reveal widespread T wave and ST-segment changes, arrhythmias (ventricular arrhythmias are common), conduction defects, particularly right bundle branch block (RBBB) or left bundle branch block (LBBB). Continuous monitoring should be commenced to monitor for these abnormalities.

Echocardiography is the cornerstone of diagnosis and will assess ventricular size and function and valvular impairment. Regular echocardiography is utilised to guide and evaluate efficacy of management. Coronary angiography should be undertaken to exclude coronary artery disease. Chest X-ray will demonstrate global dilatation of the heart and may show pulmonary oedema in heart failure.

Treatment

Initial evaluations are tailored to finding the cause, thereafter treatment is aimed at optimising cardiac function. Patients in heart failure are treated with beta-blockers, ACE inhibitors and diuretics. In patients with New York Heart Association (NYHA) III/IV heart failure, cardiac resynchronisation therapy and implantable cardioverter defibrillator (ICDs) are appropriate. In some cases, cardiac transplantation may be a suitable treatment option.

Heart blocks

Atrio-ventricular (AV) blocks, commonly referred to as heart blocks, are bradyarrhythmias resulting from AV nodal dysfunction. Interference with AV nodal conduction results in several forms of block, which may cause haemodynamic instability.

History

Heart blocks may be transient or permanent. They can arise from degenerative disease affecting the AV node associated with advancing age or from administration of pharmaceutical agents such as beta-blockers, calcium channel blockers, Digoxin and Amiodarone. Vasovagal episodes, myocardial ischaemia, inflammation or trauma resulting from cardiac surgery, such as transcutaneous aortic valve implantation (TAVI) or valve replacement, may also induce heart block.

Signs and symptoms

Patients may be asymptomatic with heart block, although bradycardia may cause fatigue, dyspnoea, pre-syncope, syncopal symptoms on exertion and hypotension. Assessment of the patient's ECG is necessary to identify and differentiate heart block.

- **1st degree AV block** (Figure 19.1): characterised by PR interval prolongation (>200 ms). QRS duration will be normal. The patient's pulse will be regular, but the rate may be normal or < 60 bpm.
- **2nd degree AV block Mobitz Type I (Wenckebach)** (Figure 19.2): characterised by progressive prolongation of the PR interval and intermittent loss of QRS complex. Pulse and ventricular rate will be irregular and usually < 60 bpm.
- **2nd degree AV Block Mobitz Type II** (Figure 19.3): characterised by a PR interval that is fixed, and often normal, and sudden loss of QRS complex.
- 2:1 block is characterised by an alternating pattern of P, QRS and T followed by a P wave which is not conducted.
- **3rd degree (complete) AV Block** (Figure 19.4): characterised by dissociated atrial and ventricular rhythms. The SA node gives rise to the regular atrial rhythm, which bears no correlation to the ventricular rhythm, which will either be a regular, normal QRS (<100 ms) rhythm at a rate of 40–60 bpm (junctional escape rhythm); or a regular, wide QRS (>100 ms) rhythm at a rate of 20–40 bpm (ventricular escape rhythm).

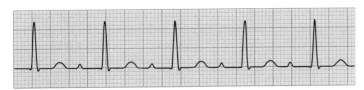

Figure 19.1 1st degree AV block.

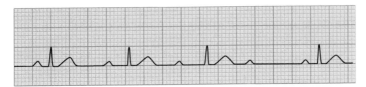

Figure 19.2 2nd degree AV block Mobitz Type I (Wenckebach).

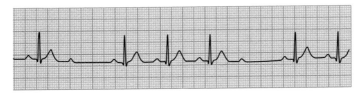

Figure 19.3 2nd degree AV block Mobitz Type II.

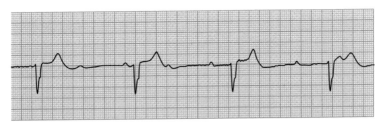

Figure 19.4 3rd degree (complete) AV block.

Assessment and investigations

Patients should be closely monitored for signs of haemodynamic compromise, including respiratory assessment, pulse, blood pressure and urine output. A 12-lead ECG should be recorded to rule out ischaemia as the cause and a history taken from the patient to establish any reversible cause of heart block.

Treatment

Patients who are tolerating heart block well should be closely monitored for signs of haemodynamic instability but may not require immediate intervention. Any reversible cause should be addressed immediately. Emergency treatment will be necessary if the patient shows signs of haemodynamic instability, usually associated with 3rd degree (complete) AV block. Atropine may be effective, particularly during vasovagal episodes, as it transiently inhibits the effect of the vagus nerve on the nodal tissue, but will be short-acting. Emergency transcutaneous pacing can rapidly augment cardiac output by increasing heart rate. However, it is likely to be very uncomfortable for the patient, hence opiate analgesia and/or sedation may be required. Insertion of a temporary transvenous pacing wire will be necessary if the bradyarrhythmia persists. Epicardial pacing may be a suitable alternative for the patient immediately following cardiac surgery. The patient may require a permanent pacemaker if the arrhythmia persists due to an irreversible cause.

Hypertension

Hypertension is known to cause coronary heart disease, stroke, heart failure, chronic kidney disease and peripheral vascular disease. It is defined as the level at which blood pressure (BP) could cause organ damage, currently established as 140/90 mmHg and 150/90 mmHg for patients over 80 years of age. Diagnosis should be made from a series of BP recordings and for treatment purposes is classified as stage 1 (>140/90 mmHg); stage 2 (>160/100 mmHg) and severe hypertension (systolic > 180 mmHg, diastolic > 110 mmHg).

History

The prevalence of hypertension is known to increase with age, although the exact cause cannot be identified in the majority of patients. Family history, insulin resistance, obesity and diabetes are strongly associated with elevated BP. Occasionally, a cause may be identified such as chronic kidney disease, thyroid or endocrine dysfunction.

Signs and symptoms

Patients with hypertension are often asymptomatic, although symptoms may manifest as a result of ensuing organ damage, such as coronary heart disease, stroke or kidney disease.

Assessment and investigations

BP should be recorded from the brachial artery when the patient is resting using either an automated device or, if the patient has an irregular rhythm, a manual sphygmomanometer and stethoscope. If the BP is found to exceed 140/90 mmHg, recordings should be taken on both arms and repeated during the consultation. The diagnosis should be made following ambulatory or home monitoring over the course of several days.

Patients diagnosed with hypertension should have their 10-year cardiovascular risk calculated as well as blood tests to establish creatinine, estimated glomerular filtration rate (eGFR), electrolytes, glucose, total cholesterol and HDL levels. A urine sample should be tested for protein, haematuria and albumin:creatinine ratio. A 12-lead ECG should be recorded and scrutinised for evidence of damage associated with chronic hypertension, such as left ventricular hypertrophy or left bundle branch block. An echocardiogram may be indicated for further investigation. Hypertension may cause retinopathy and hence the fundi should also be examined.

Treatment

Lifestyle modification is an essential element of treatment. Patients should be advised to take regular exercise and increase their dietary intake of fresh fruit and vegetables and reduce salt, saturated fat and alcohol intake. Cardiovascular risk factors, such as hyperlipidaemia, diabetes, lack of physical exercise and smoking should also be addressed.

Pharmacological therapy is indicated for all patients with stage 2 hypertension or stage 1 hypertension associated with diabetes, renal or cardiovascular disease, evidence of organ damage or a 10-year cardiovascular risk of ≥20%. Patients under the age of 55 years should be offered a once daily ACE-Inhibitor or angiotensin receptor blocker. Older patients, and those of African or Caribbean descent, should be offered a calcium channel blocker. If the response is inadequate, these treatments may be combined or supplemented with a diuretic. Specialist review may be necessary, particularly if the patient is under 40 years of age or has resistant hypertension.

If severe hypertension is found, the patient should be referred to hospital for urgent specialist review. Gradual reduction of BP over 1–2 days using oral medications such as a calcium channel blocker is necessary to avoid the risk of cerebral, renal or cardiac ischaemia, unless a specific indication, such as aortic dissection, demands more rapid BP reduction with intravenous beta-blockers or glyceryl trinitrate (GTN).

Hypertrophic cardiomyopathy

Hypertrophic cardiomyopathy (HCM) is the most common inherited cardiac disease and is the leading cause of sudden cardiac death in people under the age of 35 years in the UK. A genetic mutation results in thickened myocardium, which reduces the filling capacity of the left ventricle, inhibiting wall compliance and diastolic function, though the heart size remains normal. Syncope or pre-syncope, chest pain, heart failure and life-threatening arrhythmias may occur on exertion, although many patients remain asymptomatic and subsequently unaware of the condition.

History

HCM is caused by a genetic mutation responsible for the abnormal, chaotic arrangement of myofibrils in the ventricles that can cause arrhythmia. Significantly, this differs from the organised pattern of myofibrils seen in left ventricular hypertrophy (LVH). HCM may be identified through genetic screening of families of individuals who have the condition or who have died from sudden cardiac death. The inheritance is usually autosomal dominant.

Signs and symptoms

Patients are frequently asymptomatic with HCM although diastolic dysfunction may cause dyspnoea and other symptoms associated with heart failure. Patients may experience symptoms associated with myocardial ischaemia due to insufficient oxygenation of the enlarged ventricle, even with normal coronary arteries. Palpitations may occur due to atrial or ventricular arrhythmias. Some patients may have left ventricular outflow tract (LVOT) obstruction caused by the abnormal anterior motion of the mitral valve during systole, which may induce syncope or pre-syncopal symptoms on exertion. The first presentation may be cardiac arrest, caused by ventricular arrhythmias, most often occurring during exertion.

Assessments and investigations

Baseline observations may be normal. However, the 12-lead ECG may show increased QRS amplitude in the precordial leads, with non-specific ST-T abnormalities suggestive of LVH and 'dagger-like' Q waves in the inferior and lateral leads associated with septal hypertrophy. Cardiac auscultation may reveal a fourth heart sound or double apical pulsation caused by forceful atrial contraction into a stiffened left ventricle. Obstruction of the LVOT may be evidenced by an ejection systolic murmur heard at the left sternal border. A pansystolic murmur may be present reflecting mitral regurgitation. While the chest X-ray is usually normal in patients with HCM, the echocardiogram will provide diagnostic information. Symmetrical or asymmetrical hypertrophy of the left ventricle will be seen, along with vigorous left ventricular contraction and the systolic anterior motion of the mitral valve and subsequent regurgitation. Analysis of the family pedigree is useful to establish genetic inheritance and should be used to identify family members who may also have the condition.

Treatment

Avoiding strenuous exercise and competitive sports is strongly advised, as the increased myocardial oxygen demand and subsequent ischaemia may induce life-threatening arrhythmias. Beta blockers are usually prescribed to reduce heart rate, which will enhance diastolic function and limit the occurrence of ventricular ectopic beats. Calcium channel blockers can improve ventricular compliance. Implantable cardioverter defibrillator (ICD) implantation is recommended for prevention of cardiac arrest and some patients with LVOT obstruction may benefit from permanent pacing. Patients experiencing recurrent symptoms may be offered myomectomy or percutaneous alcohol ablation to reduce the obstructive element of the septum. Genetic counselling should be offered to all patients and family members should be screened for the condition, regardless of the presence of symptoms.

Infective endocarditis

Infective endocarditis (IE) refers to an infection of the endocardium. The condition is relatively uncommon, but can be deadly with a high mortality and morbidity. The pathological process results from endocardial injury followed by transient or persistent bacteraemia allowing bacterial adherence to the damaged surface. Infected vegetations may develop on the heart valves, which may fragment and embolise. Additionally, the heart valve and its supportive structures may become damaged, necessitating surgical replacement.

History

IE usually occurs in the presence of existing structural heart disease (valvular abnormality, prosthetic valves or congenital heart disease) and is characteristically caused by *Staphylococcus* or *Streptococcus*. It may also be due to fungal infection or as a result of drug abuse, which may cause tricuspid valve endocarditis. IE may present insidiously with the patient giving a history of a 'flu-like' illness for several weeks. Alternatively, patients may present acutely as a result of embolic events, sepsis or heart failure.

Signs and symptoms

Symptoms of IE include night sweats, malaise, weight loss and fever. Some patients may present with acute heart failure, caused by valvular regurgitation. Petechial haemorrhages in the skin, Janeway's lesions on the palm of the hands or soles of the feet, splinter haemorrhages under the nail beds or Osler's nodes, which are painful nodules on fingers or toes, probably due to vasculitis, are all extremely rare and only seen in advanced untreated endocarditis. Many patients will have a murmur on acute presentation due to valvular regurgitation.

Assessment and investigations

Careful history taking is essential to establish the diagnosis as the non-specific symptoms may mislead or confuse. Patients in high risk groups (congenital heart disease, prosthetic heart valves) who present with a fever and new heart murmur should be treated with a high index of suspicion.

Vital signs should be carried out to evaluate the temperature, heart rate and rhythm, respiratory rate and oxygen saturation. Urinalysis may reveal proteinuria or microscopic haematuria. Physical examination will include auscultation of the heart for evidence of heart murmurs. A 12-lead Electrocardiogram (ECG) should be performed and may reveal conduction defects, particularly AV-blocks or bundle branch block, suggesting development of myocardial abscess. Continuous cardiac monitoring should be commenced to observe for these conduction defects.

Physical examination may identify the features of splinter haemorrhages, Janeway's lesions or Osler's nodes. Blood cultures are a pivotal diagnostic tool and at least three blood samples should be taken at 30-minute intervals using meticulous aseptic techniques. The blood cultures will identify any causative micro-organisms although 30% of IE cases may be culture-negative. Serum blood tests will assess white blood cell count, C-reactive protein and ESR to assess for sepsis severity, urea, electrolytes, and creatinine will assess renal function as glomerulonephritis is common in acute IE.

An Echocardiogram will verify the presence of vegetations on heart valves, a Transoesophageal echocardiogram (TOE) provides better resolution and also enables assessment of structural dysfunction. Echocardiograms will evaluate the progress of the vegetations, assess for valve damage and detect abscess formation.

Treatment

In suspected IE, intravenous antibiotics should be commenced after the blood cultures have been retrieved. The majority of patients will require intravenous antibiotic therapy for 4–6 weeks and approximately 50% of patients require cardiac surgery to replace damaged valves. Patients are usually required to restrict physical activity whilst in hospital and consequently patients may become depressed because of the limitations to their lifestyle. IE is a serious condition with an in-hospital mortality rate of 20% and requires specialist cardiology care.

Long QT syndrome

Long QT syndrome (LQTS) is an inherited condition affecting the sodium and potassium ion channels of cardiac myocytes resulting in prolonged ventricular repolarisation. It can be identified on the 12-lead Electrocardiogram (ECG) as a prolonged QTc interval. Patients frequently have no symptoms but, in the event of a critically timed premature ventricular contraction (PVC), may experience the sudden onset of palpitations and syncope associated with torsades de pointes. This may deteriorate into ventricular fibrillation and therefore LQTS can potentially cause sudden death.

History

LQTS may be identified in patients with a history of cardiac events such as syncope. It can be an incidental finding on a 12-lead ECG recording or identified during a genetic screening programme. LQTS is classified by the genetic variations affecting the myocyte ion channels identified so far. The most common forms, LQT1, LQT2 and LQT3, are associated with different triggers for arrhythmia: exercise, emotion and acoustic stimuli, and rest or sleep, respectively.

Hypokalaemia, hypomagnesaemia or hypocalcaemia, bradycardia or acute myocardial infarction may cause QT prolongation, even in patients without LQTS. It can also be brought about by prolonged fasting, liquid protein diets and prescribed pharmacological treatments, such as Methadone, or specific drugs from the following groups: tricyclic anti-depressants, anti-psychotic drugs, anti-fungal agents, macrolide or quinolone antibiotics and anti-arrhythmic drugs.

Signs and symptoms

There are usually no physical signs associated with LQTS. Patients are frequently unaware of the condition until the sudden onset of palpitations and syncope, or possibly sudden death, caused by an episode of torsades de pointes. Torsades de pointes is characterised by an irregular, broad QRS tachyarrhythmia, originating in the ventricles (Figure 23.1) triggered by the occurrence of a PVC during the prolonged period of repolarisation, often referred to as the 'R on T phenomenon'.

Assessments and investigations

In the absence of arrhythmia, the QT interval can be measured on the 12-lead ECG from the beginning of the QRS complex to the end of the T wave. Broadly speaking, the R-R interval should be less than half

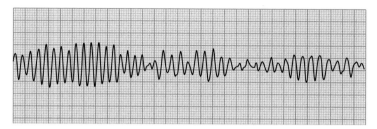

Figure 23.1 Torsades de Pointes.

the QT interval. As the QT interval is inversely proportional to heart rate, the corrected QT interval (QTc) is used for diagnostic purposes, calculated using the equation QT/√R-R interval. The QTc may be considered prolonged if greater than 440 ms in men or 460 ms in women, but often patients with LQTS have a QTc greater than 500 ms. It should be noted that short QT syndrome, another ion channelopathy similar to LQTS and Brugada, is also associated with arrhythmias.

Patients experiencing episodes of torsades de pointes will require close monitoring of respiratory function, pulse, blood pressure and continuous cardiac monitoring. 12-lead ECGs should be recorded in-between spells of the arrhythmia to establish the presence of QT interval prolongation. Previous medical history, including family and drug history, should be taken as well as blood tests, including serum potassium, calcium and magnesium.

Treatment

Torsades de pointes often self-terminates but may deteriorate into ventricular fibrillation, requiring advanced life support. Intravenous magnesium sulphate or isoprenaline may be effective, coupled with correction of electrolyte disturbance. Cardiac pacing may be beneficial to shorten the QT interval to prevent further episodes of torsades de pointes. Possible causative agents should be withheld immediately.

As there is no specific treatment for LQTS, patients are advised to avoid triggers for arrhythmia such as competitive sport, strenuous exercise, emotional distress and drugs that prolong the QT interval. Beta-blockers, cardiac pacing and implantable cardioverter defibrillator (ICD) therapy may be offered to reduce the risk of arrhythmia, although increasingly treatments vary based on the genetic type. Specialist counselling and genetic screening should be offered to the patient and their families.

Marfan syndrome

Marfan syndrome is an autosomal dominant genetic abnormality caused by mutation of the FBN-1 gene which encodes for the production of fibrillin, a protein essential for the formation of elastin fibre in connective tissue. Within the body, connective tissue provides scaffolding, anchorage and support for the skeletal, ophthalmic and cardiac systems. Abnormalities in fibrillin-1 cause the tissues to progressively stretch and weaken resulting in the potential for aortic root dissection, aortic regurgitation and mitral valve prolapse. Patients with Marfan syndrome may demonstrate a range of health problems throughout the body.

History

There may be a familial history, but 20–30% of patients present with a new mutation of the gene. Patients may be identified serendipitously when the ophthalmic (dislocation of the lens and myopia) or skeletal abnormalities (joint hypermobility, scoliosis, chest deformity or high arched palate) are identified. Marfan syndrome predominantly affects the mitral and aortic valve due to higher pressure in the left heart. Prolapse of both the mitral and aortic valves is common and may lead to mitral and aortic regurgitation. The aorta may also be affected; aortic root dilatation and dissecting aortic aneurysm are the consequence.

Signs and symptoms

There is a wide phenotype variation and those with milder forms of the disease may never be diagnosed. However, for patients with more severe forms of the condition, serious cardiac abnormality is evident. Sudden cardiac death can occur due to aortic dissection; left ventricular (LV) failure results from mitral regurgitation (MR) or aortic regurgitation. The regurgitant valves cause dilation of the LV and LA chambers predisposing the patient to arrhythmias, particularly atrial fibrillation (AF).

Assessment and investigations

Careful history taking, including familial history of sudden death, is helpful in establishing the diagnosis. Physical examination may uncover the physical features of Marfan syndrome. The Ghent criteria provide a nosology for diagnosis of the syndrome and genetic testing may identify the FBN-1 mutation. Investigations include echocardiogram and magnetic resonance imaging to assess the aortic valve size and aortic root diameter. A 12-lead ECG may identify AF or LV hypertrophy and cardiac auscultation will reveal a pan-systolic murmur in MR or an early diastolic murmur associated with aortic regurgitation.

Treatment

If Marfan syndrome is diagnosed following genetic testing, yearly follow-up and family screening is recommended. Aortic root dilatation and LV function is measured regularly using echocardiography. Beta-blockers reduce the rate of aortic root dilatation and improve survival, and the angiotensin receptor blocker (ARB) Losartan has been demonstrated to be effective, too. Medical therapy aims for a systolic blood pressure of ≤ 120 mmHg. Prophylactic aortic root and/or ascending aorta graft surgery are undertaken once the aortic root dilates to greater than 5 cm in diameter. Elective repair of aortic dissection is also undertaken to prevent sudden cardiac death. Women with a diameter of ≥ 4.5 mm are advised to avoid pregnancy without prior repair and a Caesarean section delivery may be advised. All patients with Marfan syndrome are advised to avoid exertion at maximum capacity.

Mitral regurgitation

Mitral regurgitation (MR) occurs when the valve cusps fail to fully close during ventricular systole. Leakage of blood through the valve into the left atrium results in reduced stroke volume, atrial dilatation and increased pulmonary capillary pressure, causing symptoms associated with heart failure and, frequently, atrial arrhythmias.

History

Mitral valve prolapse, age related calcification, rheumatic fever, infective endocarditis, aortic stenosis and dilated cardiomyopathy can damage the valve cusps or dilatation of the annulus, causing MR and gradual development of heart failure. The left atrium will dilate to accommodate the additional volume, often causing atrial fibrillation (AF) or flutter. Haemodynamic compensation to maintain systolic function eventually results in left ventricular enlargement. Without intervention, right ventricular (RV) failure will ultimately result from raised pulmonary and RV pressure, RV dilatation and tricuspid valve regurgitation. Acute rupture of the chordae tendineae or papillary muscles will result in severe valvular dysfunction and acute heart failure.

Signs and symptoms

Symptoms of MR arise due to heart failure. Patients may describe weakness, fatigue, breathlessness on exertion, orthopnoea and paroxysmal nocturnal dyspnoea. AF or flutter can arise from left atrial dilatation, which may additionally cause palpitations. The Electrocardiogram (ECG) may show 'p mitrale', indicating left atrial dilatation, and ECG criteria associated with left ventricular chamber enlargement. A pansystolic murmur may be heard on auscultation at the apex, with S3 and gallop rhythm. Bilateral inspiratory/expiratory wheeze and crackles may also be heard, associated with pulmonary oedema. Late signs, such as peripheral oedema, jugular venous distension (JVD) and increased abdominal girth, are associated with RV failure.

Assessment and investigations

Patient assessment should include respiration rate, depth, symmetry, use of accessory muscles and peripheral oxygen saturation levels. Following pulse and blood pressure assessment, cardiac monitoring should be commenced to observe for atrial or ventricular arrhythmias. A 12-lead ECG should be recorded to exclude acute coronary syndrome (ACS) as the cause of heart failure, to identify signs of chamber enlargement and possible myocardial ischaemia. A chest X-ray will identify pulmonary oedema and cardiomegaly if present. An echocardiogram is necessary to confirm MR as the cause of heart failure. The patient should be examined for signs of peripheral oedema, such as ankle swelling and JVD. Arterial blood gases should be taken as well as venous blood samples for urea and electrolytes (U&Es), full blood count (FBC), troponin, B-type natriuretic peptides (BNP) and glucose levels. A fluid chart should be maintained; a urinary catheter may be required to establish accurate output measurement and patient comfort.

Treatment
If the patient presents with heart failure associated with MR, oxygen therapy, diuretics and nitrates will be required. Morphine may be indicated if the patient is distressed. Supplemental treatment may be necessary for AF or flutter. Once stable, treatment should address the underlying cause where possible and aim to limit disease progression with diuretics and angiotensin-converting-enzyme inhibitors (ACE-I). Surgical repair of the mitral valve or mitral valve replacement will usually be necessary.

Mitral stenosis

Mitral stenosis occurs when calcification and fusion of the cusps reduces the diameter of the open valve. It can occur in patients with a history of rheumatic fever; most remain asymptomatic for several decades until symptoms of dyspnoea emerge. Treatment is dependent upon the severity of the condition, ranging from medical therapy to surgical replacement of the valve and annulus.

History

Mitral stenosis most frequently occurs in patients with a history of rheumatic fever in childhood, although there are other, much rarer causes. The group A β-haemolytic Streptococcus infection causes inflammation, thickening, fusion and calcification of the valvular cusps, which gradually reduces the diameter of the open valve. This limits ventricular diastole and causes a progressive rise in left atrial pressure, resulting in hypertrophy, dilatation and often atrial fibrillation (AF). Pulmonary capillary pressure subsequently increases, leading to pulmonary oedema and eventually pulmonary hypertension. Right ventricular hypertrophy and dilatation will ensue if mitral stenosis is left untreated, eventually causing tricuspid valve regurgitation.

Signs and symptoms

Patients typically experience symptoms once the valve opening has diminished from approximately 5 cm^2 to 2 cm^2, usually decades after the initial infection. The most common symptom is dyspnoea, often coupled with a cough and frothy, blood-tinged sputum associated with pulmonary oedema, caused by the raised left atrial pressure. The severity of these symptoms may worsen with episodes of AF. Eventually, elevated pulmonary pressure will cause peripheral oedema, weakness and fatigue.

The reduction in end diastolic volume causes patients to have a low volume pulse, which will be irregular if AF is present. Jugular venous distension (JVD) may occur with a prominent 'a' wave visible if the patient is in sinus rhythm. Murmurs will be evident on auscultation, usually a loud opening snap heard after the second heart sound followed by a low, rumbling mid-diastolic murmur heard best at the apex. Discolouration of both cheeks, known as malar flush, is associated with severe mitral stenosis.

Assessments and investigations

Baseline observations, cardiorespiratory assessment, chest X-ray, 12-lead Electrocardiogram (ECG) and echocardiogram are necessary to establish the diagnosis of mitral stenosis. Left atrial enlargement may be visible on the chest X-ray and seen on the ECG as a prolonged, notched P wave of > 120 ms duration (known as a bifid P wave or 'p mitrale'). The 12-lead ECG may also suggest right ventricular chamber enlargement in patients with severe mitral stenosis. These findings must be confirmed with an echocardiogram, which will establish the severity of valvular dysfunction and the extent of cardiac remodelling. Transoesophageal echocardiography (TOE) may also be used for more detailed assessment prior to percutaneous or surgical intervention.

Treatment

Symptoms associated with mild to moderate mitral stenosis may be treated with diuretics, alongside treatment for AF if required. Surgical intervention should be considered if pulmonary oedema continues, despite medical therapy or if pulmonary hypertension develops. Percutaneous trans-septal balloon valvotomy involves a balloon catheter, advanced from the femoral vein to the right atrium, where it then punctures the interatrial septum to access the left atrium and the mitral valve. The balloon is inflated to separate the cusps and then swiftly deflated and removed. Surgical valvotomy or mitral valve replacement are alternative therapeutic options that usually require cardiopulmonary bypass.

Myocarditis

Myocarditis is a life-threatening inflammatory disease affecting the myocardium. It can occur as a result of infection or from a non-infectious cause, such as sarcoidosis. The subsequent myocardial inflammation can lead to systolic dysfunction and eventually dilated cardiomyopathy, manifesting as acute heart failure, cardiogenic shock or life-threatening ventricular arrhythmias.

History

Myocarditis is most frequently caused by viral infection such as enteroviruses or Parvovirus, but can also be due to bacterial, fungal, parasitic or protozoal infection (Chagas disease). In addition to sarcoidosis, non-infectious causes include toxins, including cocaine, and autoimmune disease, such as inflammatory bowel disease.

Signs and symptoms

Diagnosis of myocarditis is notoriously difficult due to the array of clinical features associated with it, which may differ with the underlying cause. The patient may present with systemic symptoms associated with either a respiratory or gastrointestinal virus but, as the condition progresses and myocardial dysfunction ensues, chest pain, dyspnoea and other symptoms associated with heart failure may emerge.

Assessment and investigations

Patient assessment may reveal signs associated with infection and heart failure but also acute coronary syndromes (ACS), which must be rapidly ruled out. Taking a detailed history is essential as data derived from the investigations detailed below may imitate ACS. Cardiac monitoring should be commenced due to the high risk of ventricular arrhythmias and fluid balance should be closely observed.

The 12-lead Electrocardiogram (ECG) may reveal non-specific ST-T wave changes, left ventricular hypertrophy, atrial enlargement, left bundle branch block or atrial fibrillation. Cardiac troponin and B-type natriuretic peptides (BNP) are likely to be elevated along with other markers of inflammation. The echocardiogram may show wall-motion abnormalities suggestive of dilated cardiomyopathy. Cardiorespiratory auscultation may reveal signs associated with pulmonary oedema and a 3rd heart sound. Jugular venous distension may also be evident. Cardiac Magnetic Resonance imaging will enable visualisation of myocardial inflammation, oedema, necrosis and fibrosis. Endomyocardial biopsy is the gold standard diagnostic tool to enable identification of the cause of myocarditis.

Treatment

Close monitoring is essential due to the high risk of sudden death and bed rest advised to minimise myocardial exertion and to limit the extent of heart failure. Treatment for patients with myocarditis will focus on correcting arrhythmia and reducing the symptoms associated with heart failure. Drugs that might suppress ventricular contraction, such as calcium antagonists, should be avoided. Currently, no antiviral therapies for myocarditis are available. If active infection has been ruled out from the biopsy, immunosuppression therapy may be offered, particularly where non-cardiac autoimmune disease is the established cause of myocarditis. Patients may require a significant period of convalescence before returning to normal life after myocarditis, although some may not fully recover and may require cardiac transplantation.

Pericarditis

Pericarditis is an inflammatory disease of the pericardium. In one-third of cases it will also include inflammation of the myocardium, when it is labelled myopericarditis. Pericarditis generally presents acutely, although when associated with other pathology, the onset may be insidious. In most cases resolution is complete in 4–6 weeks, but in some cases recurrent or chronic pericarditis may develop. Pericarditis may occur following Acute Coronary Syndromes (ACS) and typically the patient may present 4–6 weeks after the acute coronary event.

History

The causes of pericarditis are varied and can be classified as infectious (viral, bacterial, fungal or parasitic) or non-infectious (neoplastic, metabolic, autoimmune or post-ACS). Infectious pericarditis will often present acutely with the patient giving a 2–3 week history of a 'flu-like' illness and the patient may have a fever. However, patients with a malignancy, an autoimmune or metabolic cause may present more insidiously and signs of the primary pathology may be the presenting feature.

Signs and symptoms

Classic presentation includes the following: chest pain, a fever, a pericardial friction rub, 12-lead ECG changes, evidence of a pericardial effusion and raised inflammatory markers. Chest pain is typically sharp, made worse by deep inspiration and improved by sitting up and leaning forwards. The pain is often very severe and incapacitating and the patient may be very anxious. A pericardial friction rub can be sporadic and heard over the left sternal edge with the diaphragm of the stethoscope.

Assessment and investigations

History taking is essential to establish the onset, duration and possible causes and to expedite early treatment. A detailed history of any recent infections, travel abroad or exposure to toxic substances should be carried out. Evaluation of the chest pain: onset, character, quality, duration and the factors which relieve and provoke the pain will inform the diagnosis. Typically the pain is described as continuous, sharp or pleuritic in character and widespread across the precordium. The patient may state that sitting up and leaning forward reduces the pain. A set of vital signs should be carried out to evaluate the temperature, heart rate and rhythm, respiratory rate and oxygen saturation. Physical examination may include percussion and auscultation of the lungs and heart to rule out other causes of chest pain such as respiratory infections, TB or malignancies; it may also reveal the classical pericardial friction rub. A 12-lead ECG should be performed and may reveal widespread ST-segment elevation without reciprocal ST-segment changes hence differentiating it from ACS. In addition, P-R segment depression may be seen in the acute phase of presentation, and inverted T waves may develop during the resolution phase. An Echocardiogram may establish the presence of a pericardial effusion. Serum blood tests should include full blood count, urea, electrolytes, creatinine and inflammatory markers such as C-reactive protein (CRP).

Treatment

The aim of the treatment is to alleviate the patient's pain and concomitant anxiety as quickly as possible. Opiates will not be effective in pericarditis and the mainstay of medical treatment initially is to give doses of an anti-inflammatory drug either orally or rectally to relieve the acute pain. Continued use of aspirin or non-steroidal anti-inflammatory drugs (NSAIDS) is advocated until the inflammation subsides and Colchicine may be beneficial in the long-term to prevent recurrences. The patient should be advised to rest until the symptoms resolve. Where the cause is due to systemic disease (autoimmune or renal disease, TB) or neoplasms (particularly lung and breast cancer) subsequent therapy is directed by the primary cause. Hospitalisation is only generally indicated for high risk patients or if invasive treatments are required for cardiac tamponade, large pericardial effusions, constrictive pericarditis or where cancer or metabolic disease is undiagnosed but suspected. Patients who are managed conservatively should be advised to restrict physical activity until symptom free.

Supraventricular tachycardia

Supraventricular tachycardia (SVT) is a term that describes a tachyarrhythmia arising above the ventricles at a rate greater than 150 bpm. This may include a number of tachyarrhythmias: atrial tachycardia, AV nodal re-entry tachycardia (AVNRT), AV re-entry tachycardia (AVRT), atrial flutter and junctional tachycardia. Atrial flutter and atrial fibrillation are considered separately in other chapters in this book.

History

Paroxysmal SVT is an umbrella term for any rhythm faster than 150 bpm, which originates above the ventricles. The term SVT is used when the exact mechanism cannot be identified from the surface ECG. Atrial tachycardia and A-V nodal re-entry tachycardia (AVNRT) may occur in healthy but susceptible individuals with no apparent underlying heart disease. A-V re-entry tachycardia (AVRT) is a re-entrant tachycardia associated with the Wolff-Parkinson-White (WPW) syndrome. SVTs may be precipitated by increased catecholamine or sympathetic tone, amphetamines and cocaine misuse, acid base or electrolyte imbalance, over exertion, or stimulants such as stress, alcohol or tobacco. SVTs may also be triggered by atrial and ventricular ectopics. The underlying arrhythmogenic mechanism in atrial tachycardia is enhanced automaticity; a re-entry mechanism for AVNRT and AVRT. The re-entry circuit may involve the AV node (AVNRT) or the AV node and an accessory pathway (AVRT) in WPW. The initiation of the tachycardia is generally sudden with the onset often precipitated by a premature atrial ectopic. There may be a brief period of asystole at the termination of the tachycardia. The tachycardia may last from a few seconds to several hours and may be paroxysmal, persistent or permanent.

Signs and symptoms

The tachycardia is accompanied by symptoms of palpitations, anxiety and evidence of reduced perfusion and cardiac output: dizziness, breathlessness and syncope or pre-syncope. The rapid heart rate increases the workload of the heart and also reduces diastolic filling time, hence reducing myocardial perfusion, causing chest pain and possibly precipitating heart failure and cardiogenic shock. Syncope may occur after termination of the arrhythmia due to the brief period of asystole experienced.

Assessment and investigations

Cardiac monitoring or 12-lead ECG recording will enable identification of a regular, narrow QRS complex tachycardia with a rate of between 150 and 250 bpm (Figure 29.1).

In atrial tachycardia, the rhythm arises from rapid firing of an atrial ectopic focus. P waves will be present but abnormal in morphology, R-R intervals are regular and the conduction ratio is 1:1, the ventricular rate is extremely fast, usually in the range of 140–180 bpm but can be as fast as 250 bpm, at which point AV block will develop to reduce the ventricular rate. Atrial tachycardia usually begins and ends suddenly and may occur in short bursts or be present for prolonged periods.

AVNRT is twice as common in women, may occur spontaneously or is triggered by noxious stimulants. It may also terminate suddenly or continue until medical intervention occurs. AVNRT arises due to the presence of a fast and slow conducting pathway within the AV node. In normal sinus rhythm, the impulse proceeds through the AV node, utilising the fast pathway. However, in AVNRT, if an atrial ectopic occurs early, the fast pathway is refractory and the slow pathway transmits the impulse to the ventricles. The impulse then travels backwards up the fast pathway which has recovered its excitability and this initiates a 're-entry tachycardia'. On the ECG, the ventricular rate is 140–250 bpm, and atrial impulses are either hidden within or occur after the QRS due to retrograde conduction. The QRS complex is usually narrow, unless a bundle branch block is present.

In AVRT there is a macro re-entry circuit created by the incomplete separation of the atria from the ventricles during foetal development of the heart. Abnormal collections of myocardial fibres (known as accessory pathways) are invested through the AV groove allowing a large circuit including the AV node, Bundle of His and the accessory pathway to conduct a fast reciprocating tachycardia. Patients with this anatomical abnormality, who also have symptomatic tachycardia, have a syndrome known as Wolff-Parkinson-White (WPW) syndrome. If the accessory pathway (known as the Bundle of Kent) excites the ventricles early during sinus rhythm, the excitation wave depolarises the ventricles abnormally (pre-excitation) and this manifests on the ECG

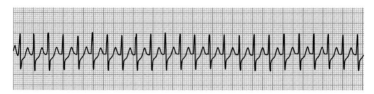

Figure 29.1 Supraventricular tachycardia (SVT).

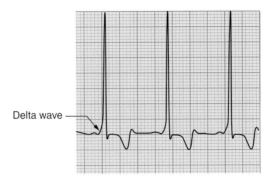

Delta wave

Figure 29.2 WPW pattern.

as a short P-R interval (due to bypass of the AV node) and a wide QRS with a slurred upstroke known as a delta wave (Figure 29.2). If a tachycardia develops, the circuit evolves from the atria to the ventricles via the AV node and enters retrogradely via the accessory pathway. This tachycardia is known as orthodromic AVRT. The tachycardia is fast, 140–180 bpm, with a narrow QRS complex (delta waves are absent), the P waves are seen after the QRS and before the T wave due to retrograde conduction.

Patients should be closely monitored for signs of haemodynamic compromise, including respiratory assessment, pulse, blood pressure and urine output. A lengthy period of tachycardia may cause cardiomyopathy and this may induce polyuria. A 12-lead ECG should be recorded and a history taken from the patient to establish any precipitant causes of the SVT and to enable differentiation of the possible type of SVT.

Treatment
In emergency situations, identification of the type of SVT may be difficult but the treatment is essentially the same. If the patient is haemodynamically stable, vagal procedures, such as the Valsalva manoeuvre may be effective. Examples include blowing into a syringe or facial immersion in cold water. Emergency treatment will be necessary if the patient shows signs of haemodynamic instability such as hypotension, pulmonary oedema or circulatory collapse. Bolus doses of intravenous adenosine will cause transitory AV block due to its short half-life, which generally terminates the SVT. Patients should be advised that the side-effects include flushing, chest pain and a sense of impending doom, but these symptoms are brief and will dispel quickly. An emergency electrical cardioversion under sedation with airway support may be necessary if the adenosine is not successful. Following resolution of the tachycardia, further investigation of causes should be undertaken and a cardiology referral made.

Takotsubo cardiomyopathy

Takotsubo cardiomyopathy (TC) is characterised by acute presentation of chest pain and/or dyspnoea due to sudden onset of left ventricular (LV) systolic dysfunction, classically triggered by an emotional or physical stressor such as anger, sadness or acute physical illness. The condition was first described in 1990 and initially it was thought that TC only affected patients of Asian origin. However, since 2003, when a Caucasian patient was noted with the syndrome, the condition is now known to be a worldwide phenomenon. In Japan, a 'tako-tsubo' is a round bottomed, narrow necked pot used to catch octopus and the shape of this pot directly mimics the LV apical ballooning seen at angiography in the presentation of this syndrome. The cause is unknown but it is thought to be due to abnormal responses to catecholamine release resulting in vasospasm and transient myocardial stunning. During coronary angiography, the patient is found to have no coronary artery occlusion, despite the presence of ST-segment elevation on the 12-lead ECG. The exact prevalence of TC is not known but there is a higher prevalence amongst post-menopausal women and hence it is suspected that oestrogens may play a role in the disease. However, TC has been observed in younger women and also in men.

History
The acute phase of TC can be life threatening and is generally triggered by an acute stressor. The onset is sudden and the patient may present in a collapsed state with chest pain and/or dyspnoea of sudden onset, which may be accompanied by arrhythmias, cardiac arrest and cardiogenic shock.

Signs and symptoms
Classically patients with TC present with symptoms similar to acute coronary syndromes (ACS) such as chest pain, dyspnoea, arrhythmias and syncope. Some patients present in cardiogenic shock or cardiac arrest. As the symptoms are identical to ACS, differentiation can only be made using angiography. The coronary arteries are found to be patent but an area of hypokinesia is present in the LV, giving rise to the characteristic 'octopus pot' shape to the LV and the potential for acute heart failure.

Assessment and investigations
The patient is likely to be very distressed on presentation and reassurance is vital. Initial assessment of vital signs should include respiratory rate, oxygen saturation and blood pressure undertaken

frequently in the initial stages. The patient should be attached to a cardiac monitor to assess heart rate and rhythm and a 12-lead ECG performed. The 12-lead ECG will be abnormal and is likely to show ST-segment elevation, particularly in the anterior leads. Importantly, there may no reciprocal ST-segment depression, which differentiates this syndrome from ACS. There may also be a prolonged QT interval, which makes patients vulnerable to ventricular arrhythmias in the recovery period.

Careful history taking is essential as a preceding emotional or physical trigger may be identified. Assessment of chest pain should elicit the duration of onset, precipitating factors, nature and radiation of pain and relieving factors. The patient may be poorly perfused with reduced capillary refill and may present in acute heart failure or cardiogenic shock.

Serum blood tests will be performed including urea and electrolytes, full blood count, clotting screen and serum markers of cardiac damage such as troponin and B-type natriuretic peptides (BNP). An urgent coronary and LV angiogram should be performed within 60 minutes of presentation, which will usually demonstrate patent coronary arteries with regional wall hypokinesia and apical LV ballooning.

Treatment

Acute management is directed towards relief of myocardial ischaemia. Opiates, such as intravenous morphine, will relieve the patient's pain and distress. Antiplatelet therapy is likely to be given in advance of the angiogram but can be discontinued when normal coronary arteries are visualised. However, anticoagulation is used to prevent stroke arising from thrombus associated with the apical dilatation. Intra-aortic balloon pump for LV support may be used if cardiogenic shock develops; diuretics are used for acute pulmonary oedema. ACE-inhibitors are used to support the LV dysfunction; most patients recover normal LV function within weeks. Beta-blockers, which inhibit the sympathetic-adrenal response to stress, may be used as prophylaxis against recurrence. Nearly all patients survive and the prognosis is good.

Ventricular tachycardia

Ventricular tachycardia (VT) is a life-threatening arrhythmia frequently associated with Acute Coronary Syndromes (ACS) that may present as cardiac arrest. On the ECG, VT appears as a series of 3 or more premature ventricular contractions (PVCs) that occur either in short salvos that terminate independently or as a sustained arrhythmia, lasting for more than 30 seconds. Monomorphic VT produces a regular tachyarrhythmia with uniform, abnormal QRS complexes that originate in the myocardium below the Bundle of His. VT can cause severe left ventricular dysfunction and may deteriorate into ventricular fibrillation (VF).

History

Patients may experience acute symptoms associated with ACS immediately prior to developing VT. Ventricular scar tissue caused by ischaemic heart disease, cardiomyopathy, myocarditis, congenital abnormalities and systemic disease, such as sarcoidosis, can permit the development of an electrical re-entry mechanism producing VT. VT may also occur in a structurally normal heart through the mechanisms of triggered activity or enhanced automaticity. VT may be due to electrolyte imbalance, particularly hypokalaemia and hypomagnesaemia, as well as the inherited ion channelopathies, such as Long QT or Brugada syndromes.

Signs and symptoms

VT is diagnosed from the ECG, which will reveal a fast, regular rhythm with abnormal but uniform QRS complexes (>100 ms) (Figure 31.1). If P waves are visible, they will not be associated with the QRS. Reduced cardiac output during an episode of sustained VT often results in hypotension, potentially causing symptoms of pre-syncope or syncope, dyspnoea, angina or reduced level of consciousness. Clinical signs include a rapid pulse (100–250 bpm) and cannon 'a' waves in the jugular vein due to atrio-ventricular (AV) dissociation. Signs associated

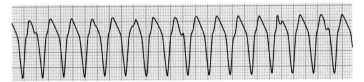

Figure 31.1 Ventricular tachycardia.

with pulmonary oedema may be evident. However, VT may be tolerated well in patients with normal left ventricular systolic function, with few signs of haemodynamic compromise.

Assessments and investigations

Patients should be rapidly and systematically assessed as VT may be life-threatening. If the patient has a pulse, continuous cardiac monitoring and regular respiratory and haemodynamic assessment, including urine output, should be conducted to closely observe for early signs of deterioration. A 12-lead ECG should be recorded and repeated once sinus rhythm has been restored to assess for myocardial ischaemia. Blood samples should include electrolytes and cardiac biomarkers to establish the cause of the arrhythmia. Regular AVPU and GCS scoring will be necessary to assess level of consciousness.

Treatment

Rapid treatment is necessary as the arrhythmia may deteriorate into VF. If the patient has already lost cardiac output (pulseless VT), advanced life support including defibrillation and airway support should be commenced. If the patient shows signs of haemodynamic compromise, such as hypotension or pulmonary oedema, synchronised electrical cardioversion may be indicated. Intravenous anti-arrhythmic drugs are suitable to restore sinus rhythm if the patient is haemodynamically stable. Identification of the cause, such as ischaemia or electrolyte imbalance, is necessary to guide the treatment to prevent recurrence. Primary percutaneous coronary intervention (P-PCI) may be indicated if ACS is suspected. Long term, an internal cardioverter defibrillator and anti-arrhythmic drug therapy should be considered as a means of reducing the risk of sudden cardiac death.

Wolff-Parkinson-White syndrome (Pre-excitation syndrome)

Wolff-Parkinson-White syndrome (WPW) is a congenital condition, which affects approximately 0.1–0.3% of the population. During foetal development of the heart, muscle strands or accessory pathways (APs) intersect the atrioventricular groove creating an extra electrical connection between the atria and the ventricles. This results in early excitation and depolarisation of the ventricular tissue. Most APs connect the atrial and ventricular myocardium at the mitral and tricuspid annuli and, as the APs may conduct either anterogradely or retrogradely, this creates a substrate for potential re-entry arrhythmias. In some patients there is a small risk of sudden cardiac death.

History

In WPW, the heart is usually structurally normal, although the APs also occur in association with serious congenital heart disease such as Ebstein's anomaly or transposition of the great vessels. The APs may conduct rapidly or slowly, bypassing the AV node, which has important decremental properties that protect the ventricles against fast atrial rates. If conduction across the AP is rapid, as in atrial fibrillation, a potential for life-threatening ventricular fibrillation (VF) may occur.

Signs and symptoms

The clinical features of WPW are variable, many patients remain asymptomatic, whilst others develop a variety of arrhythmias which may cause dizziness, syncope and palpitations causing them to seek medical assistance; in rare cases the first presentation may be due to cardiac arrest. In some patients, the ECG pattern of WPW is only discovered during routine ECG screening.

The arrhythmias associated with WPW include supraventricular tachycardia (SVT) and atrial fibrillation (AF). In the presence of AF, conduction to the ventricles via the AP causes a rapid, irregular rhythm with a widened QRS complex, which may deteriorate into VF.

Assessments and investigations

A focussed history and a 12-lead ECG form the basis of initial assessment. The 12-lead ECG will reveal a short P-R interval, less than 120 ms (reflecting the bypassing of the AV node) and a wide QRS (>100 ms) with a delta wave (Figure 32.1).

The delta wave is a slurring or widening of the proximal portion of the QRS complex, which reflects the early depolarisation of the

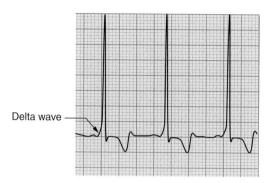

Delta wave

Figure 32.1 Characteristic ECG findings associated with WPW.

ventricular tissue. However, the remainder of the excitation to the ventricles is normal, thus the second portion of the QRS is normal. The QRS is therefore a fusion beat of early depolarisation via the AP and normal depolarisation via the His-Purkinje system. Abnormal ventricular depolarisation may produce QRS complexes of increased amplitude and there may also be ST-segment and T wave abnormalities, which may mimic conditions such as myocardial infarction, bundle branch block and chamber enlargement. Invasive diagnostic tests include electrophysiology studies to map the APs and to test the inducibility of arrhythmias.

Treatment

Emergency treatment for SVT or AF associated with WPW requires careful pharmacological management. Drugs which block AV nodal conduction such as Adenosine are not used, but Flecainide or Amiodarone may be suitable alternatives. Once back in sinus rhythm, the patient's ECG should be examined to rule out WPW as the cause. The long-term treatment for WPW depends on the degree of symptoms and the risk of sudden cardiac death. AP ablation is offered to patients considered at high risk of cardiac arrest.

Index

Rapid Cardiac Care, First Edition. Emma Menzies-Gow and Christine Spiers.
© 2018 John Wiley & Sons Ltd. Published 2018 by John Wiley & Sons Ltd.